Contents

About the authors	vii
Author's notes	viii
Introduction	1
1 You're pregnant! What now?	3
The biggest secret you'll ever keep?	3
Early symptoms	5
Getting used to being pregnant	7
Working out D-day	8
Your antenatal care	9
Scans and screening	13
The honest truth about drink and drugs	20
Signing up for antenatal classes	21
Where are you going to have the baby?	23
Going it alone	23
And the good news about being pregnant is …	24
2 Sick and tired: The joys of pregnancy	25
Ailments and symptoms – horror stories or facts?	25
First trimester	27
Second trimester	51
Third trimester	57
When to get help quickly	65
Your baby bump	68
Styling your bump	70
3 Womb with a view: Your baby's growth	73
Here's the science bit	73
How your baby grows, fortnight by fortnight	74

4 **Care instructions:** Eating, drinking, and other potentially 'dangerous' activities 86

Adapt your life, don't ditch it! 86

Alcohol 87

Cigarettes 91

Drugs 93

Caffeine 94

Food 95

Staying Zen 104

A healthy approach 104

Other 'dangerous' activities 112

Don't stop moving 117

5 **Office politics:** Pregnancy and your career 124

Your rights and responsibilities 124

Maternity leave and pay 127

Your partner's paternity rights 129

Time off for antenatal care 130

Your health and safety 130

Coping with the commute 136

If your boss is being a bugger 138

Want to go back to your career? 139

When you're the boss 141

6 **Hit and missionary:** Your pregnant love life 143

Gagging for it or just gagging? 143

Is he horny? Do you care?! 144

Make sex work 146

Bringing on labour 149

When not to have sex 150

Looking after your relationship 151

7 **Delivery schedule:** Making plans for your baby's arrival 153

Where you're going to have your baby 154

Consultant-led hospital unit 154

Midwife-led unit 155

Home birth   156
Making a birth plan   158
Hoping for a 'natural birth'?   160
Pain relief options   162
Alternative methods of pain relief   167
Your birth partner   171
The professionals   173
Birth by planned caesarean section   174
Multiple births   178
Premature birth   178

8   **Ready for take-off:** Preparing for your baby's birth   181
     The waiting game   181
     How you're going to feed your baby   182
     Shopping necessities   188
     Coping strategies for the final straight   190
     Packing your bag   196
     The things people say   199
     Your feelings   199
     Your baby's position   200

9   **Labour day(s):** What happens when you give birth   202
     You're nearly there …   203
     Going past your due date   203
     What happens when your waters break   207
     How much does it hurt?   208
     What if my baby won't wait?   211
     'Established' labour   212
     In hospital   213
     Being induced   214
     How you might act in labour   215
     Effing and blinding   216
     Here comes your baby   217
     Your baby's out!   219
     An assisted delivery   222
     Episiotomy   223

If you need an emergency caesarean   224
After the birth   225

10 Birth stories: Six *Modern Mums* recall their labour day   227

11 Hey, baby! The first few weeks with your newborn   240
Settling in   240
Feeding your baby   241
Your post-birth body   250
Recovery after a caesarean section   258
Your postnatal care   260
Baby-care essentials   262
How you'll feel   268

Useful contacts   273

Index   277

About the authors

Anya Hayes is a writer and Pilates teacher specialising in all things pregnancy and postnatal. She lives in London with her husband and two small boys. She can be found blogging at memoandjoePilates.wordpress.com, and as @anyajoeli on Instagram.

Contributing author **Hollie Smith** is a parenting author who has written 11 books, ranging from pregnancy to dealing with 'tweenagers'. She lives in Bedfordshire with her husband and two girls.

Author's notes

I've interchanged references to the baby as boy and girl throughout, and have referred to midwives as female. I've also referred to partners as 'father/dad' and 'he' throughout, but this is not to overlook the fact that other parental partnerships are legitimate nowadays. This is pure literary licence and I apologise to all male midwives and female partners.

I've included a list of useful websites and contact numbers at the back of the book, so when I refer to an organisation, look at the back for the details.

The information in this book has been checked for medical accuracy by obstetrician and mum Dr Joanna Girling.

Anya Hayes

Introduction

So, you've seen those little lines on the test confirming that you're growing a little bean in your belly. Many congratulations! You're probably feeling a mixture of exhilaration and disbelief, maybe unexpectedly shaken with a hearty dose of fear and shock? Yep. I've been there too. I've carried two little passengers around for nine months so I am well qualified to offer advice and information to help you face the next 30-something weeks of joy, fear, aches, sickness, ever-expanding girth, and everything else besides. You're building a whole new person inside you, so it's scary and brilliant at the same time. This book will expose the beautiful and the ugly side of pregnancy and be at your side all the way through, answering honestly the questions you're not sure you'd even ask your best friend.

When you're having your first baby it can feel as if you're teetering at the top of a big cliff and looking down at the unknown, about to leap off. You need the honest truth about everything that is waiting for you – not a sugar-coated version. If you're likely to develop an overwhelming aversion to your beloved clean-eating Paleo diet in favour of endless rounds of white toast; get feet the size of elephants', piles the size of grapes or fatigue which makes you feel like you're walking around in a deep sea diver's suit; it's best to be prepared – and even better to understand that these things are totally normal in the crazy, wonderful world of expecting. I'm here not only to tell you about all the medical wonders that will greet you over the course of your pregnancy, but also to prepare you for the whopping great impact on your life and make sure you're not derailed by the realities of pregnancy: juggling your high-powered career while battling unrelenting waves of nausea, and prioritising your relationship when you feel more like an elephant than a sex kitten.

Pregnancy: The Naked Truth will guide you through the ups and downs of your expectant state and the birth of your baby as honestly as possible. In other words, I'm going to tell it like it is. And, rest assured, I promise to do so without any lecturing or prescribing. Pregnancy is a time of your life when you're bombarded with advice and information, wanted or not. I'm here to guide you through and allow you to make up your own mind.

Whether you've been trying for a while to get pregnant or whether impending motherhood has come as something of a surprise, one thing's for sure: the next nine months are likely to be both exciting and terrifying in equal measure. I loved being pregnant, but I know I did utter the words 'Urrghhh I'm so SICK of being pregnant!' a fair few times while struggling to do up my shoes, or on getting a stitch if I broke into a walk marginally faster than an old lady. I have a lot more wrinkles now than I did before children. Perhaps this is due to the fact that beauty sleep is a long-lost friend of mine. But it's also because I haven't ever in my life laughed as much as I have since having babies, due to the never-ending entertainment that having children brings to your life. I look at my two beautiful boys now and I can safely say I never dwell on how rubbish I felt in the nine months I was carrying them. Think of it as a means to a wonderful end.

So, chin up. Belly out. Keep smiling. And good luck!

Anya Hayes

PS There's no better source of information on a subject than someone who's already been there and done it, which is why I've enlisted the help of a panel of *Modern Mums* who regaled me with tips and tales from their own pregnancies and births. My sincere thanks to them all for their eloquence and, above all, their honesty.

1 You're pregnant!
What now?

His sperm's hit the target. You've got a positive test result. And the excitement (or shock, depending on your initial reaction) is starting to sink in. But what now?

THE BIGGEST SECRET YOU'LL EVER KEEP?

Among the many thoughts running through your head, as you stare agog at the test in your shaking hands, is probably a desire either to shout it from the rooftops or to keep it entirely to yourself forever, as you're not sure how on earth you feel about it. First things first: it's probably a good idea to share the news with the baby's father as soon as you can, to spread the joy and panic evenly. From there, share the news with whoever you consider to be your support network. It's common to feel you have to keep schtum for the first three months until you get the 'all-clear' at the 12-week scan. But there's no law about this and it makes sense that you'd share your elation at the happy news with people you would share any emotional fallout with within that danger zone. That might be the prospective grandparents or other close relatives for bubba, or any of your good friends. Or no-one.

'I couldn't help telling people when I found out. I don't understand this obsession with keeping it secret – everyone I told I would have told if I

had a miscarriage. There's no shame or failure in miscarrying –
it's an horrific experience to go through at any stage of pregnancy,
so why is there this stigma associated with sharing such
information?'

Debbie

You may have an overwhelming urge, as I did, to tell complete random strangers on the bus to compensate for not letting the wider circle of your friends and family know until you're sure. It does sometimes feel like the most monumental secret to keep for such a long time, but it can also give you a lovely feeling of you and your partner against the world. Share as much or as little as you feel is necessary for you – it is a unique and bizarre time of your life, being pregnant for the first time, and so follow your gut about how and with whom you share.

'I felt what could only be described as … empowered. I had always
thought that I would probably feel quite apprehensive with such news,
scared of the journey and the responsibilities lying ahead, but I didn't. I
felt energised, strong, exultant and fearless.'

Beatriz

If you follow accepted tradition and keep it a complete secret until your 12-week scan, you will need some canny get-out clauses for nights out/ boozy work lunches/Christmas if you're normally the girl who likes a bucket o' wine to celebrate the end of the working week, or who is first at the bar to order a tray of espresso martinis on a girls' night out. This might be the first thing that lets the cat out of the bag (unless you're being sick 24/7, which in itself is a bit of a giveaway) – with my first pregnancy my scan date was the week after Christmas, so there was a lot of festive party-ing to be dodged, and I'm normally the person with the bottomless glass of red in her hand. FYI: drinking tonic and saying it's a gin and tonic is a win-ner, or if you're out with your partner you can adopt a clandestine system of swapping his empty glasses for your full ones … thereby meaning that he gets twice as inebriated …

You don't have to tell anyone at work for quite a long time yet. Technically, you can keep it to yourself until up to 15 weeks before you're due, although, practically, you'll probably need to spill the beans well before that – your bump is likely to start showing once you enter the second trimester, and, even before then, the fact that you keep dropping off at your desk or disappearing to the toilet every 10 minutes will probably give the game away. There's loads more about coping with work and pregnancy in Chapter 5.

'I felt like I had a big sign above my head saying I was pregnant and this huge thing was happening to me, including feeling dreadful, but amazingly no-one at work seemed to notice!'

Anna

EARLY SYMPTOMS

How it feels – and how you'll look

There's no state of being 'slightly pregnant' – you either are or you're not. Once the sperm has hit the target and the bundle of cells is on its course towards being a bundle of joy in your arms, your hormones begin on their wonderful journey too. This sets off a domino effect of changes within the body which, I'm not going to lie, can be quite weird and alarming if you normally like full control of how you look and feel. You may not even be aware of the fact that you're pregnant yet, but your body will already be trying to tell you. *Modern Mum* Lynsey said that in the week after doing the deed she noticed that all the veins in her body seemed to be suddenly very apparent and blue, which she thought was very odd until the penny dropped when she took her test three weeks later. For me, it was a very disconcerting and pronounced metallic taste in my mouth, and a feeling of being slightly and perplexingly hungover for days on end, but without a fun night out to merit it. Also, annoyingly, early pregnancy symptoms can mirror PMT feelings, so I was absolutely sure that my period was on its way and kept complaining to my husband about it. It was only when he said, after about a week of me moaning that my period was coming, 'You keep saying your period is supposed to be coming, does that mean you're late …?' D'oh!

'In a weird way I think it took a second to fully welcome something I desperately wanted, that for a long time had been something I was terrified of happening earlier in my life with the wrong person/time, etc. Though I hardly needed to worry about being a teen mum in my mid-thirties!'

Anna

Other delights include very tender and tingling breasts, a sudden and complete aversion to your usually enjoyed smells and tastes (goodbye beloved latte on the way to work), random emotional meltdowns (inexplicably breaking down in tears during Strictly). This last one sadly continues for the whole nine months and beyond, I'm afraid. Having children has meant that I can never watch Pet Rescue again.

There's a comprehensive list of what pregnancy can do to your body in the following chapter. But early signs that you've got a bun in your oven – most of them caused by the cocktail of hormones swirling around – include:

- tender, 'tingling', or slightly bigger boobs; darkening of the areola (the skin round the nipple)

- a heightened sense of smell or taste

- feeling off one or more foods or drinks, or craving something in particular

- an odd 'metallic' taste in the mouth, which is due to the surge of oestrogen in your blood

- nausea – so-called 'morning sickness' (but this is a misnomer, as you can feel sick all day or even just in the evenings) – which can kick in within days of conception

- feeling weepy and sensitive

- exhaustion and a profound heavy-legged fatigue

- needing to wee a lot

- a missed period (although you may still experience a little light bleeding, known as 'spotting', which isn't necessarily anything to worry about – see pages 28 and 66).

'I remember being very alert to smell and finding cigarette smoke utterly revolting.'

Natalie

'Because it was an IVF pregnancy I was watching for everything and yet got none of the classic symptoms initially. I was convinced it hadn't worked as I was sure I was getting my period. It was just a feeling low in my tummy, like a weight or tightness.'

Julie

GETTING USED TO BEING PREGNANT

So, your body is already on the train bound for babydom. But your mind might take a while to catch up and get on board. It is a huge thing, finding out you're pregnant – it's possibly the hugest thing that's ever happened to you. And the momentous nature of it can take its toll on your emotions, so it's important to be prepared for that. It's completely normal not to feel 100% positive about your condition, even if this is a much-wanted and precisely planned pregnancy.

The fact that the biology actually works, particularly if it's happened quickly and you've prepared yourself for it taking some time, can be a bit of a shock. Terror may take the place of elation as you realise there's no going back from this – there's no 'pause' button for your body while you get to grips with it.

'Being pregnant, or rather having a child, was something I had been desperate to do for some time, so my immediate reaction was to be ecstatic ... but almost simultaneously I felt a tremendous unease. Washing over me with increasing magnitude were waves of doubt ...

7

Was I grown up enough to have a baby? Was I selfless enough? Could I ever be responsible enough to look after a child – I had enough trouble looking after myself. An enormous weight of responsibility fell on me and I was only about six weeks pregnant.'

Nicki

Men can be a little freaked out by a positive result too (and, again, this can be regardless of the fact that they impregnated you quite knowingly). On the other hand, my husband was simply delighted that everything was working and men seem to revert into quite a primal state of being an Alpha Male, beating their chests like gorillas when it comes to this very basic level of masculinity being affirmed.

Don't feel bad if you don't feel that good about it at first. It's completely normal – most people need some time to get their head round the reality of being pregnant. Having a baby is a huge responsibility, and there's no getting away from it: your life is going to change, big time. Soon, your idea of a big night out will be falling asleep face-down in your pudding by 9pm, and a morning that starts after 6am will constitute a lie-in. But hey, it soon becomes your new normal. Reassure yourself with the knowledge that millions and millions of people have become parents before you. And have lived to tell the tale. And, more importantly, repeated it, so it can't be that bad.

'Generally I found pregnancy much tougher than I thought it would be. I thought I was quite tough and stoic, and had seen plenty of other people get on with it quietly, but when it was my turn I just felt undone! It was tiring, emotional and all-consuming. There seemed to be new things to take into account every week – new symptoms and stuff to eat or not eat.'

Julie

WORKING OUT D-DAY

Your EDD, or estimated delivery date (or your 'due date', as you'll refer to it), is a date that will loom large for the next nine months, and you might as well have it tattooed to your forehead for the number of times you'll have to answer the eager question 'When are you due?'

Your GP or midwife will work it out for you, or there are handy tools to do it online. Or, alternatively, you can work it out by counting 40 weeks from the last day of your period. This rather strangely means that when you conceive you're already two weeks pregnant. But this is based on your cycle being a regular and punctual 28 days, which not everyone's is – and, of course, it relies on you having been tracking your last period keenly. If your periods are irregular or you haven't the foggiest when the first day of your last one was, it won't be such a simple calculation – you'll be able to find out for sure when you have your first ultrasound scan and your baby's measurements will give an accurate idea of when you're due. If this differs from the date you've already worked out, it will now be the one to go by.

This highlights what a slippery science it is: try not to get too emotionally attached to your due date (although you will, as you have to tell people 78 times a day), and please remember that it is called an *estimated* delivery date because it is just that – an estimate, not a deadline or a promise. Only 5% of babies turn up when we think they're supposed to. With my first baby, I earnestly told everyone the day my baby was supposed to bounce into our lives. He took his sweet time and arrived 12 days after that date – they were the longest 12 days of my life. With my second, I offered people a very vague 'middle of January' in response to the question, and decided to see it as a 'due month' or 'two-week window' rather than a due date. This helps you to not get too caught off guard emotionally if bubs opts to surprise you two weeks early, or makes you wait for two weeks past your date, having to bat off daily 'No baby yet?!?' texts.

YOUR ANTENATAL CARE

If you haven't already, make sure you check in with a health professional at the earliest opportunity so they can make sure you get all the antenatal care you're going to need. You can go to your GP, who'll then arrange a booking-in appointment with a midwife, or you can cut out the middleman and get someone at your surgery to make this appointment for you.

Systems of antenatal care vary around the country and even according to which specific clinic, surgery or hospital you attend. The care you're offered may also be influenced by choices you've made yourself, and any risk factors that may affect you.

Responsibility for keeping an eye on you may be shared between your GP and midwife, it might be midwife- or GP-led, or, if you have any complicating factors affecting your pregnancy, a hospital-based consultant obstetrician will take charge overall, perhaps even seeing you in person during check-ups.

Some health authorities run what's called a domino scheme, where a whole team of community-based midwives look after you during your pregnancy, one of whom, in theory, will be with you during the birth, too.

You may be taking folic acid supplements already (see page 110), but, if not, it's a good idea to start popping them as soon as you know you're pregnant.

The check-ups

You'll be offered a series of antenatal check-ups with a doctor or midwife in either a clinic or GP surgery, or at the hospital. The first of these should, ideally, take place as soon as possible, some time before the 10th week of pregnancy, since some of the tests need to be carried out before then. During this initial check-up you'll be given a whole load of information, will have to answer lots of questions, and will be asked to undergo a number of tests. It's all designed to help you and your baby have good health during the pregnancy, during birth and beyond, so be as comprehensive as possible in answering and bear with all the needles and nosey questions as best you can.

It may well be the first time you've met a midwife, and you might feel a bit nervous in case she's a matronly monster, intent on telling you off for having high blood pressure and lecturing you on the evils of caffeine. The vast majority of midwives are caring (if sometimes overstretched) health professionals with your best interests at heart, and even if you end up seeing one you don't like much, chances are the one you get next time will be lovely. If you *do* have a real problem with a particular midwife, however, you may be able to arrange to avoid her in the future, by contacting either your GP or your local head of midwifery services. It's *your* pregnancy, so be confident about taking ownership of decisions like this rather than allowing yourself to feel bad or bullied by the wrong care professional.

Subsequent appointments will be much shorter and will usually involve just urine and blood pressure checks. Regular checks on the baby will also be involved. Your abdomen will be felt (you may hear the word 'palpated' used to describe this) to check his position and growth, and his heartbeat monitored. Even if you find antenatal check-ups a bit of a chore, it's always reassuring to hear the tiny heartbeat that reveals all is well. It's a good time to ask any questions or voice any concerns you may have. And don't forget to pipe up if you have any kind of health issue, or a family history of one, that could be relevant.

After about 24 weeks of pregnancy, you will usually have your bump measured at each visit. Traditionally this measurement in centimetres agrèes with the number of weeks of pregnancy. However, this doesn't allow for your size, your age or your ethnic origin. Because of this, some units have recently started to use customised charts which *do* allow for your age, BMI and ethnicity. The inventors of these charts claim that they allow better detection of babies who are smaller than they are meant to be – and this is important because they might be at increased risk of stillbirth.

Once more research has been done in this area, it will be easier to know if these charts are effective. In the meantime, keep a close eye on your baby's movements and tell your midwife the same day if they slow down. And make sure you attend all your appointments – they are really worthwhile!

According to official guidelines, antenatal appointments should take place every four weeks until you're 28 weeks pregnant, then every three weeks until 38 weeks. You should then get one at 40 weeks and after that, if you haven't yet dropped, you'll be seen at least weekly – by which time, you'll have had enough blood pressure checks to last a lifetime and will be heartily fed up with the four walls of your midwife's office. You may not have to attend them all if there are no complications. Equally, though, if anything about your pregnancy is out of the ordinary, you may be urged to present yourself more frequently.

Checking in: what to expect at your first appointment

- You'll be asked lots of questions and may have to fill in lots of forms to help create a complete picture of your health (and your partner's), family history, work and lifestyle – all things that may in some way affect you, your pregnancy or your baby.

- You'll be asked about where you want to have your baby.

- You'll be weighed, measured, and have your BMI calculated. Your midwife needs to know if you're significantly overweight or underweight, as these could prove complicating factors.

- You'll be asked for a urine sample (as you will on all subsequent check-ups, so you'll get used to weeing into a funnel). This can help doctors detect a number of potential problems, such as pre-eclampsia (after 20 weeks, see page 41).

- Your blood pressure will be taken (and at every subsequent check-up). It's common for blood pressure to rise in pregnancy and it's important to keep tabs on it because if it gets too high it's another sign of pre-eclampsia.

- A number of blood samples will be taken, to establish your blood group and to check for iron-deficiency anaemia (see page 30) and for a number of infections which, while uncommon, could cause a problem for you or for your baby.

- You'll be given lots of other information about looking after yourself and the baby, the further tests and scans that you'll be offered, and your choices regarding your antenatal care and the birth.

You may well get to the end of your first appointment wondering if you're having a baby or applying for a job at NASA. It's a lot to take on board – still, at least you've got about another eight months or so to digest it.

Your antenatal notes

All pregnant women get their own personal set of antenatal notes – you'll usually be asked to keep hold of them yourself in between appointments, so you'll need to take care to bring them back for the next one, and to take them with you if you go on a trip away, just in case of a medical emergency. Do try your best not to leave them on the bus.

The notes will usually contain useful telephone numbers, and advice on what to do if anything concerns you.

If you're bewildered or concerned about the battery of tests, scans and screening that you're offered during your pregnancy, don't worry – you're not alone. To add to the confusion, not all the available antenatal tests are routinely offered in all areas, so make sure you know what you can get.

SCANS AND SCREENING

Thanks to the marvels of modern technology, you'll get at least one chance to see your baby before he's born, via an ultrasound scan. For most prospective parents, this first, fuzzy glimpse of their little alien offspring is a proud and thrilling moment – even if all you can ever really make out is a jelly-like blob which bears little resemblance to anything human.

According to guidelines from the National Institute for Health and Care Excellence (NICE), you *should* be offered two routine ultrasound scans during your pregnancy, including one at some point between 10 and 13 weeks, usually known as the 12-week or dating scan.

Smile, please

Most hospitals will let you take away a printout of your scan images, usually making a small charge of three or four quid. This cherished memento will give you your first chance to bore other people with your baby pictures – just don't expect them to be as excited as you are by the sight of the grainy, nondescript blob that's your son or daughter.

You may have heard about 3D and 4D scans, which provide an uncannily detailed image of your baby. You definitely won't get one of these scans on the NHS, so if you're keen to have one, you need to contact a specialist service, of which there is a growing number these days.

A dating scan means your docs can firm up your EDD – or establish one, if you haven't been sure until now – by taking the baby's measurements. It will also reveal how many babies you've got in there.

Obviously, in most cases, it's just the one – but around 15 in every 1,000 pregnancies result in twins, and about 150 women a year receive the gobsmacking news that they've scored a hat-trick and conceived triplets. Depending on the policy of your hospital, you may also be offered nuchal translucency screening during this scan (see below).

In spite of the fact that every pregnant woman ought to get a dating scan on the NHS, there are still a few pockets of the country where they are not offered routinely. Some couples who find themselves in this position choose to have one done privately for peace of mind, usually at a cost of around £100 to £150.

Whether or not you get a dating scan, you should certainly be offered one at around 20–22 weeks, by which time it's possible to see the baby in a bit more detail. This one is known as an anomaly or mid-pregnancy scan, and is used to detect any abnormalities in the baby (although it's not guaranteed to pick up every potential problem) and to check that all's well with her growth and position. The sonographer – the trained professional who carries out scans – will usually point out any visible bits of interest, like the baby's spine, and her heart, which you'll be able to see beating. You'll probably be able to make out the outline of her face, and pinpoint one or both of her hands and feet.

If anything's out of the ordinary, you may be offered more scans than usual. And if there's something doctors want to keep an eye on, such as a low-lying placenta (see below), you should be offered at least one more scan, later on in pregnancy, to check that it's moved up.

Medical factfile: a low-lying placenta

Sometimes the placenta – the amazing organ that acts as a life support system to your baby by passing on oxygen and blood from you – implants low in the uterus and ends up covering, or at least threatening to cover, the cervix (the entrance to the womb). Usually, a low-lying placenta will move out of the way later on in pregnancy, in plenty of time for your baby to be born. But in about 10% of cases it won't and it then becomes known as a placenta praevia. This is a potentially risky condition, since it can cause severe bleeding, and your medical team will want to keep a close eye on you. If it's largely, or completely, blocking your baby's exit route, you'll almost certainly need to have your baby by planned caesarean section (see page 174).

Does it hurt?

Scans should be painless for you and your baby, but, depending on the skill of the sonographer and the position of your baby, you may experience some discomfort as they try to locate the information they need. You'll need to present yourself with a full (but not too full) bladder, as it can help push up your womb and so give a clearer picture. Given the average waiting time in a busy antenatal clinic, combined with the already dysfunctional state of most pregnant women's bladders, this can make for a pretty uncomfortable wait beforehand.

The other slight unpleasantness is the gel that's wiped across your naked tummy to help the probe glide across: it's bloody freezing.

Sonographers tend to work in silence, concentrating on seeking out all the baby's bits and on taking measurements. This can seem a little ominous, but it's normal. They'll talk you through what they can see once they're done.

Boy or girl?

Increasingly these days, it's common to find out the baby's sex at the anomaly scan. Lots of parents-to-be want to know whether their bundle is a boy or a girl – perhaps because they want to decorate and shop accordingly, decide for definite on a name, or feel it will give them a head start on the bonding process. Of course, some people are still keen for a surprise when it comes to their baby's gender and don't feel the need to know. If this is the case, though, be warned: you'll be fending off the question, 'Do you know what it is yet?' until the day when you finally do.

If you *do* want to know whether it's a girl or a boy, bear in mind that you may not be offered this information automatically, and might have to request it – pipe up at the beginning rather than the end of the scan, so there's time for the sonographer to look. There are still some hospitals where the policy is not to let on, usually because they can't guarantee it will be accurate. If they refuse and you simply *have* to know, you might consider going private. On the flip side, as it is so common nowadays to find out, you may have to tell your sonographer early in your scan that you *don't* want to find out, to avoid them letting it slip accidentally, as, for them, it's sometimes very obvious (even though to us it all looks like swirly snowstorm nothingness).

Remember, no-one can give a 100% guarantee of an accurate answer to this question. Once in a while, an umbilical cord gets mistaken for a willy and little Johnny turns out to be a Jane. The website of the Foetal Anomaly Screening Programme is a good source of further information about scans.

Testing for Down's syndrome

These days, all pregnant women are offered some form of testing for Down's syndrome, a chromosomal abnormality that affects about one in every thousand babies born each year. Your risk of having a baby with Down's increases as you get older – from approximately one in 1,500 for women of 20, to one in 900 for women of 30, to one in 100 for women of 40. Testing for Down's is completely optional, and some couples don't feel the need. However, if tests establish that you *do* have a baby with Down's, you'll have time to weigh up your options – or even just to prepare for the emotional and practical needs of a child with this condition.

Initially, you'll be offered screening which won't tell you for sure whether your baby has Down's, but will indicate whether you're at high risk or not – only around 3% of tests will throw up a high-risk result, and remember, it doesn't mean for certain that your baby has Down's syndrome. Likewise, if you get a low-risk result, that doesn't mean there is no risk at all.

Screening to show the risk of Down's syndrome is done by blood test, or by ultrasound (when it's known as a nuchal translucency scan, or NT), or most commonly and accurately by a combination of both. Which type you are offered will depend on what the policy is in your area – some couples also choose to go private at this point. There is a new, more accurate blood test that used to be only available privately but has been offered in NHS teaching hospitals as part of a research programme over the past couple of years. More recently, this has been rolled out generally in a few areas for women at the time of their dating scan. This test is also known as the NIPT non-invasive prenatal test and is available privately if your hospital doesn't currently offer it, and, in combination with the evidence presented at your scan, it is said to be more than 99% accurate at predicting a risk of Down's, but less so for Edwards and Patau syndromes. There is a slight wait for the results of this test – up to two weeks of nervous waiting for a phone call – whereas the others you receive on the day of your scan.

If you do get a high-risk result from this initial screening, you'll be offered a diagnostic test, which will give a more definitive answer, but carries with it a slight risk of miscarriage. If it comes to this, you should get lots of support and information, as weighing up whether or not to take this option can be a tricky one. But in the end it's a personal decision, and one that only you, and your partner, can make.

There are two types of these tests available: amniocentesis and chorionic villus sampling (CVS). Amniocentesis involves having a scan to check the position of the baby, and a fine needle being inserted into the womb to take a sample of amniotic fluid, which can then be tested. CVS is a similar process but involves taking a sample of placental tissue, rather than fluid. Both procedures cause some discomfort.

An amnio certainly isn't a pleasant thing to go through. 'It didn't hurt exactly, but it's very invasive – physically and emotionally,' reveals *Modern Mum* Alison. 'I glanced at the monitor only to see this enormous needle go past my son's head, which made me feel a bit giddy. It was all over before I knew it.'

On average, there's a 1% chance of miscarriage being caused by amniocentesis, and a 1%–2% chance with CVS – a risk you'll probably want to weigh up carefully before going ahead. 'There was a high risk of my son having Down's, which was why I was offered an amnio,' explains Alison. 'I blubbed for several hours, saying there was no way I would willingly have a procedure that carried a risk of miscarriage. But after the consultant explained that the risk varied from hospital to hospital, and theirs was much lower than average, I went ahead. In the end I was glad I did. The result was negative, and it meant I could relax and enjoy the rest of the pregnancy.'

You may have to wait up to a week or more for the results, and, happily, in the majority of cases they'll be negative. But if the result is a positive one, you should be offered all the advice and support you need to decide what happens next.

Medical factfile: Down's syndrome

- Named after John Langdon Down, the doctor who first identified it, Down's syndrome is a genetic disorder that affects around one in 1,000 babies.

- A baby born with Down's is likely to have a low birth weight and a number of typical features that include slanting eyes and a flat back to the head. Physical symptoms include floppy joints and poor muscle tone. There's also an increased risk of problems with sight, hearing, heart and digestive systems.

- Children with Down's usually develop at a slower pace than other children, and will have some degree of learning difficulties.

- There's no cure for Down's syndrome, but lots of support and treatment is available that can improve health and quality of life.

When there's a problem

The majority of tests taken during pregnancy reveal all is well. But sometimes a significant problem or potential problem is detected, which can be worrying, even devastating. Should you need them, a charity called Antenatal Results and Choices (ARC) exists specifically to help people through this experience.

The test you won't get as a matter of course

Group B Streptococcus (Group B Strep or GBS) is a common bacterium that's carried in the vagina by around a quarter of pregnant women, usually harmlessly. However, it can be passed on from mum to baby during birth and occasionally this causes very serious problems. According to the charity Group B Strep Support, 75 babies die every year from neonatal GBS, and 40 are left with long-term health problems.

GBS can be picked up incidentally during other antenatal tests and, if this happens, you'll be offered antibiotics during labour (which means that your labour is now classed as one that needs intervention, so you won't be able to have a home birth), as this measure can significantly reduce the chances of your baby picking up the infection.

However, many women won't know if they're carriers or not, as screening for GBS is not carried out routinely in this country. It's not screened for mainly because the test itself is not 100% reliable, and you can have 'flare-ups' of GBS and only test positive for it at certain times, which means you may be positive at 16 weeks pregnant but not necessarily at 32 weeks. Campaigners recommend that women consider taking a test themselves through one of several private labs that offer this service. There's lots more information on the website of Group B Strep Support.

THE HONEST TRUTH ABOUT DRINK AND DRUGS

Unless you've been very cautious and given up drinking in preparation for becoming pregnant, chances are you've been continuing with life as normal and find out you're pregnant when you're already a few weeks gone. This might mean that your usual Friday night post-work drinks, Saturday brunch hair of the dog … and Tuesday evening cocktails … have been continuing unimpeded by the knowledge that you're preggers. You might feel immediately guilty for drinking before you found out, but please don't worry. Just stop the benders now!

I got very drunk before I knew. Could it have harmed the baby?

It's very unlikely. And if you didn't actually know you were pregnant when you downed all that Pinot Grigio, there's not much you can do about it, so there's definitely no point in beating yourself up.

Plenty of women have found themselves in this position – in fact, let's face it, large numbers of babies wouldn't even have been conceived if it weren't for heavy drinking sessions. Chances are you'll have caused no harm at all, although clearly it's a good idea to ease up on the drinking once you do know. However, there's nothing stopping you from sensibly enjoying the odd alcoholic beverage or two if it's something you enjoy (see page 87).

'The week before I did the test I had an impromptu work night out, in the pub until 2am drinking beer, wine, shots ... maybe subconsciously I knew it might be the last time for a while. But when I did the test I thought, SHIT, what have I done? I decided not to freak out but just not to touch any more alcohol for the rest of my pregnancy.'

Vicki

What about drugs?

Different drugs have different risks, but whatever it was, a one-off session is unlikely to have harmed your baby. Don't take any more though. If you have a real problem in this area, tell your midwife and get yourself and your baby the help you need. There's more on the subject on page 93.

SIGNING UP FOR ANTENATAL CLASSES

A word to the wise: if you think you'd like to join the National Childbirth Trust (NCT) and sign up for their antenatal classes, do so now. NCT classes are beloved by middle-class mummies-to-be everywhere, and consequently tend to fill up quicker than you can say 'natural birth' – so make contact with your local branch sooner rather than later if you're interested.

If you can't get into an NCT class, or can't afford to pay (fees start at around £120, depending on where you live, although there are opportunities for subsidies), your midwife or doctor will tell you about the NHS classes available in your area, probably a bit nearer your due date. (There is also a growing number of private antenatal options, many run by independent midwives and involving luxury weekends away in classy hotels – lush, if you can afford it.)

NHS antenatal classes, often called parentcraft classes, are run by midwives and are usually pretty basic. Their availability and scheduling can also be a bit hit and miss, as they tend to be subject to funding and staff cuts.

NCT classes, on the other hand, are run by specially trained teachers and take place in small group settings, sometimes in the teacher's home, which all lends it a very intimate feel. It depends on the mindset of the teacher, but you might notice a distinct bias among NCT types towards natural birth and breastfeeding, which, for many, is an unwelcome pressure. I was lucky and had an NCT teacher who had experienced all types of birth herself – she had first had an emergency caesarean, then a hospital vaginal birth, then a home birth, and was amazing and open-minded and reiterated constantly that all birth is a valid birth experience, which is ultimately what you need from antenatal classes. But this may not always be the case.

More importantly, though, if you attend a local class you're going to meet other prospective parents there, and while you're bound to run into at least one other person who makes you want to stab yourself in the eyeballs, you've got a good chance of running into some like-minded folk. You may even forge some long-term friendships. There is a slight pressure to meet your 'best friends forever' through NCT groups. Some people do, some people don't. However, whichever antenatal class you choose, there is something very valuable in having a small group to go through this very intense and unique journey of first-time parenthood with, and it means you will have people you can text at 3am when your baby is two weeks old and you're not sure if their poo is a normal colour.

'In my NCT group there were six couples, and five of us ended up having a caesarean. We all felt like all the discussion of natural birth seemed slightly pointless in hindsight! It was a great way to meet a group of people to go through this exciting time with, though.'

Debbie

There are pros and cons to all varieties of antenatal classes, but in most cases they're a practical way to get information and to help you prepare emotionally and practically for the birth. In particular, they can be a good way to get your man interested – up until later pregnancy he may feel slightly detached from your growing baby, as it's growing in your belly not his, after all. Antenatal classes can make this impending new human much more 'real' and imminent for dad. A bit of a kick up the arse, if you like.

WHERE ARE YOU GOING TO HAVE THE BABY?

You'll be asked early on to think about where you'd like to have the baby, and informed of what your choices are where you live. (You're entitled to go out of your area, though, if you feel strongly about it for some reason.) Once you've decided, your doctor or midwife will 'book you in' at the unit of your choice. But you don't have to make this decision in a hurry if you don't want to – and when you do, you can still change your mind about it later in pregnancy. There are three main choices:

- a consultant-led hospital maternity unit

- a midwife-led birthing centre, if there's one in your area

- a home birth.

There's more about the pros and cons of each in Chapter 7.

GOING IT ALONE

It may have taken two of you to get pregnant, but sometimes only one of you is around to see the pregnancy through. If you're on your own (or in an unstable relationship, and likely to be that way before very long), you may be feeling even more anxious about what the future holds. Chances are you're in for a slightly harder than average pregnancy – all the difficulties, but with no-one there to support you through them. As single mum Kemi testifies, 'I knew it would be really tough and I have to admit I was terrified when I realised I'd be going it alone, but I knew that I would have a lovely little strong team, just me and my baby.'

Now's the time to draw on the support of anyone else around you who cares from among your family and friends, so that you never have to go to a scan on your own and at least there'll always be someone at the end of a phone to commiserate if you feel sick, tired or scared. There are also lots of organisations and websites that offer information, advice and friendship – it's worth checking them out.

AND THE GOOD NEWS ABOUT BEING PREGNANT IS …

If all the early symptoms, reams of information, endless questions, and emotional ups and downs you're going through are getting you down, maybe it's time to remind yourself that your pregnancy is in fact a wonderful thing. Need a few more reasons to be cheerful? How about these?

- No periods for a while. Yay!

- No contraception needed, either.

- More likelihood of a seat while using public transport. (Well, once you're big enough for people to be sure they're not insulting you before offering, that is ….)

- Free dental treatment. Make sure you get a check-up.

- People are genuinely really nice to you and you get a lot more smiles and joy sent in your direction. (Warning: strangers will want to touch your belly.)

- You really need to take it easy and you certainly shouldn't be exposing your baby to all those chemicals in cleaning products … what a shame.

- Great knockers. For the poorly endowed among us, the upgrade from A to B or more is definitely a bonus.

- You're going to need an extra 200–300 calories a day to keep your strength up in the last trimester.

2 Sick and tired

The joys of pregnancy

AILMENTS AND SYMPTOMS – HORROR STORIES OR FACTS?

Before we launch into a list of the various discomforts you can look forward to over the next few months, I want to first remind you of one of the most noted benefits of pregnancy that all of my *Modern Mums* picked up on – when you're pregnant, pretty much everyone is friendly to you, even when you don't really want them to be, like when you're on the bus feeling grumpy in the rain on a Monday morning. It's a lovely sense of joy that your growing belly seems to bring to your surrounding area, like you're spreading a cloak of sugar sprinkles around the world. Even on the greyest, most uncomfortable of days, there will often be someone who makes you feel pretty special for doing this ordinary but extraordinary thing of baking a new small person in your oven.

'I got treated like a special gem within my family. My boyfriend looked after me even more than he usually did, strangers in the street looked after me, everyone just acted like I was a precious, delicate thing, which I was really unused to. I liked it!'

Hannah

So now let's talk about what pregnancy will mean for your body, other than the obvious big belly stuff. You should steel yourself for some fairly brutal truths here – pregnancy may not be an illness, but it sure does have a lot of weird and wonderful symptoms. A massive release of hormones is to blame for most of them, coupled with the obvious physical strain of nourishing and carrying the bub. Ironically, your options for medication are limited because of potential risks to the baby, and, in many cases, no-one's found an effective treatment anyway. So pregnant women are generally expected to grin and bear whatever they're dealt. (Although I suspect that if *men* were responsible for gestation, someone would have invented a cure for morning sickness by now.)

'Imagine waking up with a horrific hangover EVERY morning. You end up eating carbs like they are going out of fashion even though you know that it is a myth you can "eat for two" and every morsel of those snacks your body is craving is going straight to your thighs.'

Becca

As a very general rule, you can expect most of the really crap symptoms to strike during the first trimester, when the pregnancy hormones are at their most active, and in the third, as the ever-expanding passenger inside you grows, kicks, grows, presses, and grows some more in the final stretch. The second trimester is the one in which all the so-called 'blooming' is supposed to take place, and certainly most women report it to be the most enjoyable bit.

Of course, different women experience different pregnancies. You may get off lightly and suffer nothing more than a handful of minor irritations. Or you may have ticked off the whole back catalogue by the time your nine months are up. It's all down to luck, genetics … and hormones.

But try to keep some perspective: as *Modern Mum* Clemmie says, 'When you look back it's hard to remember what all the fuss was about, but at the time it was utterly hellish!' Keep this in mind if you're overwhelmed by feeling uncomfortable some days. This too shall pass, and your body will one day be yours again (albeit slightly altered!).

Here, then, is a comprehensive list of the delights that can crop up during pregnancy, trimester by trimester. I've listed the symptoms when they may first appear, although some can, fantastically, be experienced throughout pregnancy. Be assured that these are all normal niggles (as obscure as some may seem) and, in themselves, are *usually* nothing to worry about – however much grief they're giving you. Where they *might* signal something more serious, I've said so. Follow your gut – if you ever feel like something's not quite right, always call your midwife just to be sure.

Word of warning

If you're in any doubt at all about something your body's doing which it didn't do before, ask your midwife or GP. Don't feel embarrassed or silly because you want to know why your nose is bleeding, your bottom's hurting, or your veins are protruding. They're used to it. If you need an answer quickly and it can't wait, try 24-hour 111.

There are some symptoms which you should seek advice on urgently: see page 65.

FIRST TRIMESTER

Abdominal pain

What is it and why is it happening?

It's not unusual to feel pains of one sort or another in your tummy throughout the whole of your pregnancy. Although worrying, they usually don't signal a major problem. Early on, there can be a little period-like pain as the embryo implants in your womb. A sharp, stabbing pain in the side or groin is common in the last trimester, and it's common to get a stitch if you're moving too fast, but this is likely to be nothing more than the stretching of the muscles and ligaments around the uterus. You may also suffer the delights of constipation (see page 35), or wind (see page 56), which can be quite uncomfortable. From the second trimester onward, and particularly as you reach the final stretch, it's common to feel 'practice' contractions known as Braxton Hicks, which can cause some pain or discomfort (see page 203).

'The worst thing was the stretching pains. I got really upset and worried that something was wrong. I went to A&E and they said I needed an early pregnancy scan. Once I had it they told me everything was fine and the pains soon passed.'

Jo

What can I do about it?

It depends on the cause, but not very much. It will probably help if you can sit down and get some rest.

Could it be serious?

Generally speaking, tummy pains are only a cause for concern if they are prolonged, or very severe, and/or you have some other symptom alongside them, such as regular, rhythmic tightening of your abdomen, bleeding, a high temperature, chills, vomiting, blood in the urine or pain urinating. If the pain becomes more severe over time, you must see your doctor. Early on in the first trimester, the pain could be a sign of an ectopic pregnancy (see box below) and it's imperative you seek help if the pains are severe as this can be life-threatening. It's always possible that abdominal pain is caused by something not related to your pregnancy, such as appendicitis, which your doctor may need to rule out. Or it could simply be that you've been eating too much chocolate.

Bleeding in the first trimester

Bleeding in the first trimester, before your first scan, may be nothing to worry about, as some spotting is common when the egg implants itself into your uterus wall. However, always keep a close eye on it and consult your doctor if you are worried. There can be more serious causes which you do need to be aware of, including ectopic pregnancy (when the egg has started to grow outside the uterine cavity, most usually in the fallopian tubes), molar pregnancy (a very rare complication which means the fertilised egg doesn't develop into an embryo, or develops abnormally and can't survive), or a miscarriage.

Miscarriage is something that doesn't get talked about enough, in my view. Although absolutely devastating, it is sadly common, occurring in up to one in four (recognised) pregnancies, most of those in the first trimester. I've had three miscarriages, but I've also had two healthy babies. So for me, personally, miscarriage is intertwined with my experience of pregnancy, as I have spent many months with five pregnancies, disguising those first weeks of pregnancy grottiness, only for it to end in sadness three times. You have to bid farewell to all those plans, hopes, visions, dreams that you inevitably create the minute you see that positive pregnancy test. I know how heartbreaking it is, it is truly crap. Usually, and perplexingly, there's no reason and nothing you can usefully blame – in the vast majority of cases, it's nature's way of dispelling a fetus that has a problem. But that knowledge doesn't really help when you have to pick yourself up afterwards.

It's worth bearing in mind that the experience of miscarriage will possibly have a bearing on your mental health throughout subsequent pregnancies, with heightened levels of anxiety being common. It is important to remember that many, many women go through this and possibly just don't ever speak about it. So, my advice: speak about it if you want to, and certainly talk to your GP if you feel that you're often feeling low or struggling to cope. Once you do, you will realise how many people understand and have been through it too. This is one reason why I've sworn off ever asking anyone about their 'plans to have a baby', you simply don't know what they're going through with their fertility journey and it's not worth pressing a wound without realising. If it has happened to you, or someone close to you, be mindful of your/their mental health. Women in this situation need to be encouraged to look after themselves, physically and mentally; they will need time for their bodies to recover, and time to grieve. If you are pregnant and are worried about a friend who has had a miscarriage, don't be a stranger. They will be truly happy for you and your bump; it may just be tinged with some pain, particularly around due dates and anniversaries. So be patient and kind to them. You can get help and more information from the Miscarriage Association. Details are at the back of the book.

Anaemia

What is it and why is it happening?

In most cases, anaemia during pregnancy is caused by iron deficiency, which pregnant women are more prone to because of the increasing demands on their blood supply. The lack of iron means a decrease in blood cells, leading to symptoms such as exhaustion, palpitations, headaches, dizziness and shortness of breath. It can also make you more prone to infections. This can affect you at any stage in your pregnancy. Your baby's brain also needs a good supply of iron for optimal development.

What can I do about it?

The best way to fight anaemia is by making sure you eat plenty of foods that are rich in iron (see page 110). Your GP or midwife, who'll be alert to the possibility of anaemia and may pick it up during a routine antenatal check, could suggest you take iron tablets. These often have an unwanted side effect – constipation – and you may have to try more than one sort before finding a type that suits you. There are various iron supplements you can take, and most pregnancy supplements contain additional iron. Be careful to ensure that any supplements you take are cleared for pregnant women, and check with your GP if you're at all uncertain.

Could it be serious?

In most cases anaemia won't be a major problem, although it can make you feel pretty poorly and exhausted. However, severe anaemia may mean you are more likely to need a blood transfusion if you have a postpartum haemorrhage (see page 221), so your midwife or doctor might want to investigate further.

Anxiety

What is it and why is it happening?

We've all heard of 'postnatal depression' and it looms large in the imagination as a scary 'thing' that happens after the baby arrives. Increasingly being recognised, though, is the fact that heightened levels of anxiety or low feelings during pregnancy can increase the risk of developing postnatal depression. Figures released in 2015 by the Royal College of Midwives suggest that up to 20% of women experience perinatal mental illness during pregnancy and in the first year of their babies' lives. It's particularly common if you've struggled with fertility issues, or have had recurrent miscarriages. The new pregnancy guidelines published by NICE for healthcare professionals suggest that there should be 'screening questions' asked at regular pregnancy checks, to look out for warning signs, and support should be offered where needed.

This is different from regular healthy 'worry' – you'd have to be slightly unusual to sail through pregnancy without ever freaking out about your growing baby, your life ahead, the birth, running out of chocolate digestives … No, this is where normal worry tips into something that starts to control your life in a negative way and needs to be managed. The Maternal Mental Health Alliance describes perinatal depression and anxiety as including constant symptoms such as 'tumble-dryer mind', insomnia, feeling tense and irritable, social paranoia, shakiness, blurred sight, racing heart and breathlessness. If you recognise these symptoms in yourself, chat to your midwife or GP, and don't suffer in silence.

‘I was surprised by how I seemed to change from being relatively easy-going to suddenly very fearful and jittery about everything. I spoke to my midwife about it and apparently it's quite normal. My GP referred me for a course of CBT [cognitive behavioural therapy] to try and deal with it before it became serious.’

Kelly

What can I do about it?

Share the load and talk to someone about it. It takes confidence to speak up, but try not to feel scared to admit to feeling less than ecstatic if it's clear that you're feeling low or anxious most of the time. Even if you're not able to confide in your partner or midwife, acknowledge to yourself how you're feeling and try to incorporate managing techniques into your pregnancy – take a regular yoga or mindfulness class, or allow yourself some pampering time. Anything that reduces tension in the body will help to calm the mind. If you feel happy to, ask to be referred for counselling, which can give you some tools to keep your mental health on an upward trajectory.

‘I did worry about how parenthood would affect me. I'm not a fan of uncertainty, and in lots of ways your first pregnancy is one of the most uncertain times of your life!’

Natalie

Could it be serious?

If left unchecked, perinatal depression can lead to postnatal depression, so it's really worth nipping heightened anxiety in the bud. You don't want it to mar the first months of enjoyment of your baby's life.

'Baby brain'

What is it and why is it happening?

Does something happen to women's brains to make them more forgetful during pregnancy – or do they just have a lot on their mind? Science hasn't come up with an answer yet, but anecdotal evidence suggests that as many as half of pregnant women suffer from 'baby brain', or 'preg head' as it's sometimes known. This can be a problem throughout your pregnancy, and beyond ....

What can I do about it?

Nothing – other than writing yourself lots of lists and keeping calm about it. Remind your partner that it is an actual 'thing', and if necessary leave this book open at this paragraph so he understands and doesn't say anything uncaring.

Could it be serious?

No. (Not unless one of the things you forget is to turn the gas off, or something else potentially lethal.) There's a bit about coping with 'baby brain' at work on page 136.

Bigger, tender boobs

What is it and why is it happening?

Changing hormones, increasing blood flow and the beginnings of milk production all contribute to bigger boobs in the first trimester. This can be good or bad news, depending on how big they were in the first place – and, unfortunately, the increase in size is often accompanied by tenderness and discomfort. Later in your pregnancy, you may also experience a little leakage of colostrum (the creamy, first phase of milk production). You might as well get used to this – your boobs are going to fill up to bursting point after the birth and a bit of leaking now is just the start.

What can I do about it?

- Get yourself fitted for a new bra. Chances are you've gone up by at least a cup size so go for something as comfortable and practical as you can bear. A good bra will also help minimise sagging – an inevitable downward trend for many women.

- Get measured several times during pregnancy as your assets may swell by up to three cup sizes overall.

- If you're really big or in a lot of discomfort, you might want to wear a soft cotton sleep bra at night, too.

- A little gentle massage can ease tenderness – on the other hand, some women can't bear even to be touched.

Could it be serious?

Only for your other half – such a beauteous bounty, and strictly not for him when they're sore.

Bleeding gums

What is it and why is it happening?

Changing hormone levels cause the gums to swell and become more sensitive than usual and, in some cases, this can lead to soreness and bleeding – known as gingivitis.

What can I do about it?

- Pay careful attention to your dental care to minimise plaque, which can make the problem worse.

- Brush your teeth and gums twice daily with a fluoride toothpaste for at least two minutes (even if it makes them bleed more); don't forget to floss.

- There are a couple of mouthwashes on the market that claim to help – your dentist should be able to recommend an appropriate one.

Could it be serious?

If left untreated, gingivitis can cause major decay to teeth and gums. And that won't be anything to smile about.

Smile, it's free

Don't forget that NHS dental care is free when you're pregnant, so make the most of it. You can get the exemption form you need from your midwife or GP reception.

Breathlessness

What is it and why is it happening?

Many women find they're struggling to catch their breath at some point during pregnancy. It's very normal, and it occurs because your lungs are having to work harder to provide extra oxygen; also, later in pregnancy, your growing uterus pushes against your diaphragm, the muscle that helps control breathing.

What can I do about it?

Not a lot. It's normal and harmless, but if an attack of breathlessness occurs, don't panic. Try to sit down and rest for a while.

Could it be serious?

Not usually, although it can be a sign of anaemia if it persists (see page 30), or other things like a chest infection or blood clot in the lung (pulmonary embolism), and you should let your midwife know if you're experiencing any other symptoms as well, such as palpitations, chest pain or coughing up blood.

Constipation

What is it and why is it happening?

Problems with pooing commonly happen for two reasons during pregnancy: hormones relax the digestive system, which slows down the movement of food through it, and your growing uterus puts pressure on your bowels and bottom. It's particularly likely to affect you if you're prone to it anyway, or if morning sickness is preventing you from getting a balanced diet.

'The constipation in those first three months was horrendous,' recalls *Modern Mum* Alex. 'I was reduced to taking fig tablets, which would ultimately result in emergency dashes to the loo. It was most unpleasant.'

What can I do about it?

● Eat plenty of fibre-rich foods such as wholemeal bread, fruit, vegetables and pulses – and, crucially, drink lots of water to help it all move through.

- Regular gentle exercise such as walking, yoga and swimming.

- Constipation is a common side effect of iron tablets, so if you're taking these for anaemia try cutting them out or switching brand.

- If things get really bad, a gentle laxative treatment may help, but be sure to get advice or a prescription from your doctor or midwife as some laxatives are too strong for safe use in pregnancy.

Could it be serious?

No, although it can make you seriously miserable if you've also got piles.

Cramps

What is it and why is it happening?

Cramps are sudden spasms of pain in the legs and feet. It's not clear why they can crop up during pregnancy, but theories include muscle fatigue (other muscles in the body are working so hard to support you and the growing baby, and something has to give); a deficiency of minerals such as magnesium and potassium; and pressure on the nerves caused by the growing uterus.

What can I do about it?

- Try not to cross your legs when sitting or standing; keep your legs and ankles moving by stretching and wiggling your calves and feet whenever you get a chance.

- If you do get an attack, stretch out the leg and rotate your ankle, or try walking round the room.

- Gently rubbing the muscle can help.

- Eating a balanced diet may help boost any minerals you're missing – bananas are a great source of potassium if you can stomach them, but check with your midwife or GP before taking any type of supplement.

Could it be serious?

No, just annoying. They'll only come in short, temporary bursts and won't last beyond pregnancy. If you've got severe, persistent leg pain and/or you're suffering from other symptoms such as swelling of the leg, contact your GP as this could be a sign of a deep vein thrombosis (see below).

Medical factfile: thrombosis

Around one or two in every 1,000 women will get a blood clot in the vein during pregnancy or just after birth, when the risk is about five times higher than normal because of changes in the way the blood clots and flows. (And some people are more at risk of blood clots in general because of a genetic tendency, so you should always let your midwife or doctor know early on if it's something that runs in your family.)

The most common sort – deep vein thrombosis (DVT) – is when a blood clot occurs in a deep vein, usually in the leg. Symptoms include pain, tenderness and swelling in the leg, which may turn pale blue or reddish-purple in colour. If you notice any of these, alert your midwife or doctor immediately. All women are risk-assessed for DVT in pregnancy and at delivery.

Treatment is a medication called heparin, which is safe for your baby and doesn't affect breastfeeding. You may be asked to inject yourself once a day with heparin to stop a clot forming. This might be during pregnancy, after birth or both. You could also be asked to wear compression stockings to improve blood flow and reduce swelling. It's vital to get prompt treatment for DVT, as it can lead to a dangerous complication called a pulmonary embolism, which can prove fatal.

Exhaustion

What is it and why is it happening?

This is one element that comes as a shock to a lot of first-time mums-to-be. The fatigue in the first trimester can make you feel like you've been hit by a freight train. Think about the alchemy that your body is undertaking in that first three months – whirring up an entire new human out of a ball of teeny tiny cells, setting in place all the organs, creating the body parts – and even though your body may not have visibly changed yet, you'll begin to understand why you're so goddamn tired all the time. Later on in your pregnancy, the sheer hard work involved in carrying all that extra weight can also make you very tired. Towards the end, you could be lugging around the equivalent of up to seven bags of sugar (baby, uterus, placenta and amniotic fluid included). It can then be compounded by other common features of pregnancy such as insomnia, nausea, poor diet or a lack of exercise. Exhaustion can be a symptom of anaemia, too; so if you're really struggling, you should chat to your midwife about it and have your iron levels checked.

'The body-slamming tiredness of the first trimester was unexpected. I didn't understand all the things that my body was doing and wasn't prepared for how completely exhausted I would feel. I fully expected to be tired in the last few months, as by then I would be hauling around a lot of extra weight, but in the first three months there was no outwardly physical change that could account for how I was feeling.'

Nicki

What can I do about it?

Not much, other than resting as much as possible, getting in as many early nights as you can, and enlisting your partner or someone else to take charge of housework and the like. You've got a great excuse, so indulge your inner granny and go to bed early and put your feet up.

'The worst thing was the absolute, superlative, beyond this world, exhaustion. For six weeks within that first trimester, I was unable to stand for longer than 10 minutes. Or raise my arms and wash my hair. I felt a level of tiredness that I had neither experienced nor envisaged. I just had this feeling of life abandoning me. It felt like I was slowly and relentlessly losing all my energy.'

Beatriz

Could it be serious?

No. Not unless you fall asleep in a dangerous place …

Food cravings and aversions

What is it and why is it happening?

Pregnancy cravings are the subject of many a joke. They're very real though. For *Modern Mum* Melissa it was oranges and chilli con carne, for Zoe it was smoked mackerel and pineapple. Some women also go off certain foods, most usually caffeine, alcohol, and anything greasy or spicy. It's not really clear why either of these things happen although there's a theory that they may be an evolutionary mechanism, helping to ensure that a pregnant woman gets what she needs.

What can I do about it?

Most cravings are harmless and can be indulged, although if you're living on a diet consisting entirely of cold baked beans or chocolate Hobnobs as a result, you should probably aim to rein it in for the good of your health.

Could it be serious?

Craving a non-food item is a psychological disorder known as pica and, unsurprisingly, it isn't a good idea to consume something that's, frankly, inedible.

Among the weird items pregnant women have been known to hanker for are sand, coal, soil, soap, sponges, cigarette butts, matches, plaster, mud, sandpaper and rubber – and you don't need me to tell you that none of these are good nutritional options. A yearning to chow down on a non-edible item may be more to do with texture than taste, so you might be able to get some relief from chewing on something crunchy but innocuous, like ice.

Hairiness

What is it and why is it happening?

Thanks to those lovely old hormonal fluctuations, you may find that you have increased hair growth during pregnancy: usually a bonus on your head (where it may also appear greasy, or, if you're lucky, shinier than usual) but rather less desirable over the rest of your face and body. However, some women find it works the other way and they have less body hair, or that some of the hair on their head falls out.

What can I do about it?

Up the ante on your usual depilatory regime – waxing, plucking and shaving are all fine, but do a patch test before using a hair removal cream, as skin tends to be more sensitive during pregnancy. Although there's no evidence that electrolysis and laser treatment can be harmful to a baby, some practitioners advise against it.

That said, you might find you're better off relaxing about hairier body parts – let's face it, pregnancy is one of the few times in your life when you can get away with being fat, spotty and hairy. In any case, have you ever *tried* waxing your bikini line with a 38-week bump?

Could it be serious?

Er, no. (BTW, there's no truth in the pregnancy myth that a hairy belly means you're having a boy.)

Headaches

What is it and why is it happening?

Frequent headaches are another of those common pregnancy symptoms where the cause isn't really understood. Hormones and the change in blood supply are probable culprits, and other factors including nausea and dehydration, nasal congestion, insomnia and stress may also play a part. I suffered worst in the first trimester but headaches can strike in all three.

What can I do about it?

- If you're suffering from a headache, or can feel one coming on, try to find a moment to lie down, preferably in the dark, and rest. A lavender head cushion or cooling eye mask works wonders.

- Doctors generally advise against any sort of medication in pregnancy; aspirin and ibuprofen are out, but moderate doses of paracetamol are okay.
- If you're prone to headaches, aim for prevention rather than cure by getting as much sleep and rest as possible, eating well and drinking plenty of fluids.
- Caffeine is probably best avoided.

Could it be serious?

If you're getting many, or severe headaches or migraines, or you're having other symptoms alongside them such as blurred vision, vomiting or swelling, do mention it to your midwife as there's a chance they could indicate pre-eclampsia (see below).

Medical factfile: pre-eclampsia

Raised blood pressure is very common in pregnancy, but up to one in 10 women will develop pre-eclampsia, a potentially serious form of pregnancy-related high blood pressure in which there is usually also protein in the urine and sometimes the baby is smaller than expected. It will develop only after 20 weeks and is likely to be detected during routine antenatal tests on your blood pressure and urine. Because of the risks of pre-eclampsia, you'll be closely monitored if you're found to have high blood pressure at any stage.

Symptoms of pre-eclampsia may include headaches, swelling in the hands and feet, blurred vision and vomiting, but not many people experience them.

If you are diagnosed with pre-eclampsia you are likely to be advised to stay in hospital since in one or two out of every 100 women, it has serious risks and can become dangerous for you or the baby. It can cause some potentially fatal complications for you, including eclampsia (convulsions), stroke, kidney failure, liver damage, and the breakdown of the body's blood-clotting system; and for the baby, abruption (bleeding behind the placenta), intrauterine growth restriction (IUGR) and, in some cases, intrauterine death.

You may be offered medication which can reduce your blood pressure. But the only cure for pre-eclampsia is to deliver the baby.

All of which is why you're likely to be admitted to hospital so you and your baby can be carefully monitored and an early delivery arranged if necessary.

Mood swings

What is it and why is it happening?

As your nearest and dearest will no doubt vouch, your mood during pregnancy can be, well, changeable. Contrary to popular opinion, it's not necessarily a time of rosy glows and permanent smiles, and it's totally normal to feel intermittently miserable, since those rampaging hormones take their toll emotionally as well as physically. Naturally, you may also be worried or anxious about many things. And, let's face it, if you're feeling like death thanks to the nausea, backache, or any of the other delightful symptoms outlined elsewhere in this chapter, it's just going to make things worse.

What can I do about it?

Keep your chin up: mood swings may frequently punctuate the first trimester but will usually subside once you get into the second, and only resurface towards the end. Meanwhile, try to get as much rest and sleep as you can, and look for distractions in whatever makes you happy: a good book or movie, some relaxation exercises, or an evening with friends. Talk about it if you can, preferably to someone who's good at listening.

Could it be serious?

A certain amount of mood swinging is very normal, but perinatal depression (see Anxiety, page 31) is an issue that healthcare professionals are becoming more aware of. It's known that women who feel very down during pregnancy are at higher risk of developing postnatal depression after the birth, so if you're feeling particularly low for prolonged periods, chat to your midwife or GP – they may refer you for counselling, or prescribe a safe form of medication.

'I've always done a good line in crying at silly things but that definitely increases in pregnancy. I found myself sobbing at the song *You've Got a Friend in Me* earlier this week.'

Julia

Morning sickness

What is it and why is it happening?

Nausea is experienced by as many as 85% of pregnant women. It usually starts by around week six of pregnancy and can last up to around week 15, or for some it magically disappears once past the 12-week mark. 'Morning sickness' is a stupid name, as it very often lasts all day, or is just in the afternoon and evening. For some women it involves actual vomiting, while for others it goes no further than the distinct feeling that they're just about to. And it's horrible because it's so relentless, often going on without any let-up for days, weeks and even months, like the longest and worst hangover you've ever had. For me personally, it was a distinct but low-level sickie feeling that became worse in the evening. I got off lightly – *Modern Mum* Julie was throwing up every single day for 16 weeks, poor thing ...

'The nausea: praying to the porcelain god at 6am, naked, crying and dry heaving. I was lucky enough to have full-blown sickness only a handful of times but I felt really nauseous whenever I was hungry (which was constantly).'

Jenn

'My first trimester was pretty rotten – from five weeks till about 14 weeks I felt constantly sick. I wasn't actually sick at all, but I felt horrid. Vegetables, in particular, were revolting – the smell, texture, taste. I survived on toast and satsumas as everything else made me feel like vomiting.'

Bella

Doctors aren't really sure what causes it, although inevitably those fluctuating hormones generally get the blame. There's also an evolutionary theory: sickness is nature's way of putting pregnant women off potentially harmful foods. Either way, it can be one of the worst elements of early pregnancy, especially when it's accompanied by other symptoms such as exhaustion. Appetite is often affected; in fact, some women find they can't face food at all – and then worry about the lack of nutrition their baby is getting.

Morning sickness won't harm your baby, who'll still thrive even if you eat nothing but ginger nuts and mashed potato for three months. The good news is that it usually eases up once the first trimester is over. Morning sickness is also believed to indicate high levels of the hormone human chorionic gonadotrophin (hCG) – it's this that nourishes your baby until the placenta takes over the job at around 12 weeks and so there's an unproven theory that morning sickness is a sign that all is well with the pregnancy. (Please note, though, that this is no reason to fret if you *aren't* experiencing morning sickness – not all women do.)

'The constant sickness and puking was absolutely horrific. I have always been a sickie person. Especially on a hangover. So to feel that way every day made me weak. I would want to weep at the prospect of getting onto a packed tube full of smelly people (my sense of smell was suddenly on a par with a blood hound), holding myself back from retching until I was in a safe environment. You keep reminding yourself you're not ill – you're pregnant – but sometimes it's hard to spot the difference.'

Becca

What can I do about it?

- Try to keep eating if you can (easier said than done) – little and often, if you can't face full meals. Experiment to try to find things that you can stomach – anything spicy or greasy is best avoided. Things that have worked for others are toast, digestive biscuits, crisps and cereal.

- If you can't eat at all, remember to drink instead to avoid dehydration – especially if you are actually vomiting. Some women find flat cola does the trick.

- Ginger is an alternative remedy that is reckoned to help – try nibbling ginger biscuits, or drinking hot water infused with real ginger root.

- You could try an acupressure band, worn round the wrist, which is said to relieve nausea by pushing down on a particular pressure point. They're available from larger chemists and health food shops.

Could it be serious?

Only when it's hyperemesis gravidarum (see below), which is what our dear princess Kate Middleton suffered from in both her pregnancies, leading to the pregnancies being revealed to the world by the media very early on, as she was hospitalised at around six weeks with the first pregnancy. It is hard to hide something as severe as that. It's also important to seek help if you have vomiting that's accompanied by other symptoms, such as fever or pain, in case it's being caused by a completely different medical problem.

Medical factfile: hyperemesis gravidarum

Excessive vomiting in pregnancy is known as hyperemesis gravidarum. Although it's not harmful for your baby, it can cause severe dehydration that may lead to hospital treatment and, often, some weight loss. It can be really miserable, particularly as it's often passed off as ordinary pregnancy nausea and therefore 'just one of those things'. However, it's important to seek out a sympathetic health professional if you're suffering, as treatment is available in the form of anti-sickness

---

medication. With modern and pre-emptive treatment, intravenous fluids and anti-sickness medication can be administered as an out-patient, so hospital admission can usually be avoided.

Pelvic pain

What is it and why is it happening?

Thanks to the release of the hormone relaxin, the pelvic joints loosen in pregnancy to allow room for the baby's exit. Unfortunately, this increased mobility causes discomfort and/or pain in the pelvic region as well as in the buttocks, hips, legs and lower back for many women. There may also be an audible clicking or grinding sound when you move. This condition is widely known as pregnancy-related pelvic girdle pain or PGP. It can strike at any point in pregnancy and sometimes just afterwards. Usually, the first trimester and third trimester are the problem areas.

What can I do about it?

- Keep gently active – avoid resting, as this weakens the muscles which are trying to support your pelvis, and mean that you have too much time for thinking! But avoid the activities that hurt.

- Pay attention to your posture: aim to keep your knees close together and, when standing, try to keep straight so your weight is evenly distributed over both legs. If you love swimming, avoid breast stroke as the action of the legs will exacerbate pelvic pain.

- If PGP is causing significant discomfort or pain, your doctor may pre-scribe painkillers, or refer you to a physiotherapist who will suggest exercises that can help and who can provide equipment such as a pelvic support belt or crutches – or even a wheelchair, if necessary.

- Pilates exercises can be a great help, although make sure you go to a pregnancy class with a qualified practitioner who has been trained to deal with prenatal issues; just attending a regular class at the gym could make things worse.

- Some women report that alternative treatments such as osteopathy provide considerable relief, so you might want to consider looking at private practitioners if you're not getting much relief from your NHS team.

Could it be serious?

For some women, PGP can become so severe it makes ordinary activities such as walking, making love and even turning over in bed agony. PGP can also have implications for the birth and for caring for your baby afterwards, since the symptoms can continue after pregnancy. In these cases, a referral for physiotherapy will be vital. A related condition, diastasis symphysis pubis (DSP), occurs when an abnormally large gap develops between the two pubic bones at the front of the pelvis. If you need more information on pelvic girdle pain, we've included some useful addresses at the back of the book.

'I had PGP and by the end I couldn't walk any longer than five minutes without being in agony – I even resorted to being pushed around in a wheelchair when I needed to go Christmas shopping!'

Debbie

Restless leg syndrome

What is it and why is it happening?

Restless leg syndrome (RLS) can affect anyone at any time, but doctors are unclear about its cause and why it is more common during pregnancy. It's described as an uncomfortable, sometimes painful, urge to move the legs and a feeling that your legs are 'tingling', 'crawling' or 'burning'. It usually strikes when you're resting, especially at the end of the day, so it's most likely to occur when you're sitting down in the evening or lying in bed. Symptoms are usually eased by moving or massaging the legs but return again when you're resting – naturally, it can make it hard to get to sleep.

'I'd be sitting on the sofa with my partner watching TV and trying to relax, my legs resting on his lap, when I'd have to jiggle them around as if I had ants in my pants. He always thought I was being weird but there's no way of describing it, you just HAVE to move your legs around!'

Julia

What can I do about it?

Standard advice is to cut out alcohol and caffeine and aim to relax in the evenings – measures you're probably taking in any case. You could try using a pregnancy pillow to support your body while resting and sleeping. Other than that there's little you can do, unfortunately; do try to keep busy as this can distract you from the uncomfortable symptoms.

Could it be serious?

No – and like so many irritants of pregnancy, it will magically cease once you've had your baby.

Sensitivity to smells

What is it and why is it happening?

This is mainly a first trimester issue, but it can last for the entire pregnancy for some. Many pregnant women report that their sense of smell becomes very acute and that certain things (very often husbands) are suddenly emitting a pungent whiff: 'I made my partner change his aftershave as his usual one made me queasy, but then the first time he wore the fairly expensive one I made him buy as a replacement, I was nearly sick,' reveals *Modern Mum* Anna. It's thought that this could be down to the same rush of hormones that (probably) causes morning sickness – and, as with morning sickness, there's also a theory that it's an evolutionary thing, in place to help pregnant women automatically veer away from bad or potentially poisonous foods.

What can I do about it?

Nothing, really. If you ask your husband nicely, he will perhaps agree to station himself in another room – for the time being anyway.

Could it be serious?

No, although your other half could end up with hurt feelings.

Thrush

What is it and why is it happening?

During pregnancy, the natural balance of bacteria in the vagina is affected by hormones, which means you're up to 10 times more likely to get thrush: a yeast infection that causes a thick, creamy discharge and soreness or intense itching in and around the vagina.

What can I do about it?

- Eating natural yoghurt is said to keep thrush at bay because it contains infection-busting organisms – you can also apply it directly on your bits for some soothing (if messy) relief.

- Anti-fungal creams and pessaries are available on prescription or over the counter – some thrush treatments aren't suitable during pregnancy though, so check with your doctor or the pharmacist first.

- Avoid wearing tights and tight trousers, and only wear cotton pants.

- Avoid perfumed shower gels and soaps, which make the irritation worse.

- Don't forget that your partner may also need treatment in the form of cream, as thrush can be passed on sexually.

Could it be serious?

No, although it can get you down, especially if it keeps coming back.

Urinating (lots)

What is it and why is it happening?

Feeling the urge to wee a lot more is a symptom that can kick in early on in pregnancy – because of hormone changes, and because there's a lot more fluid in the body generally during pregnancy, as the kidneys step up a gear to rid the body of waste products.

Wee-wee overdrive usually eases up after the first trimester but often returns with a vengeance later, due to the growing pressure on the bladder caused by your expanding womb.

This is often another reason for those disturbed nights. 'Every night I have to get up at least once to go to the loo,' says *Modern Mum* Kate, 'but I know that this is probably training for broken sleep once baby comes so I guess it's good practice.'

What can I do about it?

Not much.

- Don't be tempted to hold it in – always go with the flow, as it were.
- Make sure you've always got access to a loo – plan your journeys accordingly.
- Aim to totally empty your bladder each time you pee, by 'rocking' back-wards and forwards on the toilet a little.
- Don't be tempted to stop drinking, as we all need lots of fluids to keep us healthy – although you could try reducing or cutting your intake late in the evening to avoid a disturbed night.
- Avoid or cut down on anything containing caffeine as it has a diuretic effect (that is, it encourages urine flow).

Could it be serious?

Not in itself, but be wary of symptoms such as bloody or cloudy wee, or pain when urinating, which could signal a urinary tract infection (UTI). It's really important to get UTIs diagnosed and treated as they're a trigger factor for premature labour (see page 178).

Vaginal discharge

What is it and why is it happening?

It's normal to have more vaginal discharge than usual during pregnancy – driven by your hormones, it's nature's way of helping to protect against infections that could travel up you to your uterus. It could also be a sign of cervical ectropion (see the box on bleeding in pregnancy on page 66). Late in pregnancy you may get a thick 'show' of discharge which could include some blood – this is a sign that labour is imminent (see page 203).

What can I do about it?

Nothing, there's no need. Avoid washing with perfumed soaps or shower gels and never douche (that is, forcefully aim a jet of water up there) as it can upset the balance of chemicals in the vagina and increase your risk of infection. If it's really heavy, you can always wear a panty liner (never a tampon, for the same reason).

Could it be serious?

Keep an eye on any heavy discharge – if it becomes dark in colour or smells odd, mention it to your midwife or GP, in case you've got some kind of infection. A watery discharge in late pregnancy should definitely be reported: it could be leaking amniotic fluid, which could signal premature rupture of the membranes (see page 179).

SECOND TRIMESTER

Itching

What is it and why is it happening?

Mild itching is normal and is caused because of the increased blood flow to the skin, and also as the skin stretches across your growing belly. Because it's generally associated with skin stretching as your baby grows bigger, this condition is more likely to occur from the second trimester onwards. Pregnancy hormones also make the skin more sensitive than usual, and therefore more prone generally to rashes and itchy patches.

'I had a peculiarly itchy belly (my bump). SERIOUSLY itchy. The midwife thought I developed eczema on my belly because of how much my skin had to stretch (for an 8 pound baby). It went away immediately after birth. It was so itchy I used to literally look forward to getting home from work so I could put my feet up and do nothing other than scratch my belly! It drove my husband mad watching me scratching all the time.'

Claire

What can I do about it?

Wear loose clothing made of natural fibres, and try using a gentle, soothing cream such as calamine lotion.

Can it be serious?

Severe itching, particularly in unusual places such as on the palms of your hands or soles of the feet, can occasionally indicate a potentially serious liver condition called obstetric cholestasis (see below), so keep your midwife informed.

Medical factfile: obstetric cholestasis

It's not clear what causes obstetric cholestasis, a liver disorder that leads to a leakage of bile salts into the bloodstream.

The most common symptom, which usually doesn't develop until the third trimester, is itching; sometimes mild, sometimes unbearable, and often worst on the hands and feet. The condition can also cause tiredness, mild jaundice, dark urine and a lack of appetite. Because studies in the past have linked the condition with an increased risk of stillbirth, women who are diagnosed with obstetric cholestasis are closely monitored and usually offered an induction at 37 or 38 weeks.

Obstetric cholestasis is purely pregnancy-related and will cease to be a problem once your baby is born.

Nosebleeds and nasal congestion

What is it and why is it happening?

The increased blood supply experienced in pregnancy, driven by your hormones, puts pressure on the veins inside the nose and causes the sinuses to swell, which makes them more prone to bleeding and/or nasal congestion (as well as snoring). Nosebleeds can be alarming if you've never suffered from them before, but they're completely normal in pregnancy. As *Modern Mum* Charlotte reveals: 'Throughout my whole pregnancy I had a stuffy nose and sounded like I was suffering from a cold.' For me, the nasal congestion was worse at night-time. My husband told me that my pregnancy snoring made him feel like he was sharing a bed with a family of bears.

What can I do about it?

- If your nose bleeds, remain upright and pinch it gently but firmly for up to 10 minutes, which should stop the flow – if not, repeat.

- Take care to blow your nose gently when you need to.

- Stuffiness can be relieved with a little steam inhalation. Fill a sink with hot water, cover your head with a towel and take a few deep breaths. I kept an over-the-counter decongestant inhaler by the bed and used it whenever my breathing was getting difficult. Check with your GP or pharmacist, or carefully read the label of all decongestants, before using, to check that it's safe during pregnancy.

- If it gets bad, your doctor may prescribe a safe decongestant.

Could it be serious?

It's likely to be a harmless annoyance. However, frequent or heavy nosebleeds can cause anaemia, so if they're bad, seek help.

Pain in the hands

What is it and why is it happening?

One of the slightly weirder side effects of pregnancy is carpal tunnel syndrome (CTS), and it's caused by a build-up of fluid in the tube that houses the wrist nerves. It leads to variable levels of pain, throbbing, numbness or pins and needles in the hands and fingers, and it commonly gets worse at night. If severe, it can affect your ability to carry out everyday tasks.

What can I do about it?

Resting and raising the hands as much as possible can help. If you're really suffering, you should be referred to a physiotherapist, who may recommend wrist splints and can give you some exercises that will help.

Could it be serious?

In most cases it eases after the baby is born. Occasionally it persists and a minor surgical procedure is needed.

‘Somewhere around month five, I began waking up in the night with an intense pain in my hands, almost as if they were put to sleep with razors. Describing this as "pins and needles" would be a gross understatement as my hands felt massive and painfully numb. I would reach for my glass of water on my night stand with what felt like Frankenstein's hands. It would take about 10 to 15 minutes (feeling like hours) of me shaking and clenching my hands for the pain to subside. I eventually had to wear wrist guards in the evenings as well as to sleep, which helped but didn't completely stop the insanity.’

Jenn

Skin changes

What is it and why is it happening?

All sorts of odd things can happen to your skin because of hormonal changes. Changes in pigmentation can cause dark patches on the face – or, if you're dark skinned, lighter patches – sometimes called 'the mask of pregnancy'. This can happen at any stage in pregnancy, but usually appears from the second trimester onwards.

For the same reason you may also notice moles, freckles, birthmarks and your areolas (the skin around the nipple) darkening, and the appearance of a dark line running down the centre of your tummy – known as the 'linea nigra'.

Increased levels of blood can make your skin appear rosier than usual (hence the alleged 'blooming' or 'glowing' of women during pregnancy) and can also sometimes lead to the appearance of spider veins – small clusters of broken capillaries on the face and body. Some women find they get spotty, since hormones drive an increased production of sebum, the oily substance that keeps our skin supple.

You may also notice the appearance of skin tags, harmless blobs of excess skin that can appear anywhere on the face or body.

What can I do about it?

Not much. Most skin changes don't cause any harm, although they may look unsightly, and they will fade back to normal after pregnancy. You could cover up patches, spider veins and high colour with a good foundation, and tackle oiliness with a really thorough cleansing regime.

Could it be serious?

No. It will probably be the least of your worries. If any moles do change shape, size or colour drastically, though, get them checked out by your GP.

Varicose veins

What is it and why is it happening?

Swollen, bulgy veins that cause pain or itching are a common feature of pregnancy, as the hormones cause the blood vessels to relax and the body's increased blood flow and growing uterus put pressure on your veins. They're most common on the legs, in the anus (where they're better known as piles, see page 62) and inside the vagina. Being overweight and hereditary factors can increase your chance of suffering from them. Women carrying multiples are also more at risk.

What can I do about it?

- Put your feet up – literally. If you're suffering from swollen or aching veins in any part of your body, keeping your legs up whenever possible can help ease the pressure.

- Make sure you get regular rests if you need to stand up for work (for more on your rights at work, see Chapter 5).

- Support tights or stockings can offer some relief, while for vulval varicosities there's something on the market called a v-brace, like a rather large pair of padded support pants.

- An ice pack (or bag of frozen peas) may prove soothing.

- It's sensible to exercise gently and keep active, to boost your circulation.

Could it be serious?

No, just painful and unsightly. They'll usually go away or go down at some point after the baby's born. If not, and if they're severe, it's possible to have surgery to remove them.

Wind

What is it and why is it happening?

Bet you never thought you'd give your man a run for his money on the farting front, did you? Well, now's your chance. All those extra hormones can play havoc with a pregnant woman's digestive system – compounded later on by the pressure of the growing uterus on the stomach – and, as well as constipation and indigestion, one of the end results of this is an increase in bloating and wind. Lovely!

What can I do about it?

- Specific foods can make things worse, so you could try pinpointing the usual suspects and removing them from your diet.

- Eat small meals, and take care to chew your food before swallowing.

- Keeping active can help, too.

Could it be serious?

No. But your other half might object to the fact that you now burp more than he does.

THIRD TRIMESTER

Back pain

What is it and why is it happening?

Ever seen a heavily pregnant woman push her hands into the small of her back and wince? Back pain affects as many as three-quarters of women in pregnancy. Hormones again. This time it's something called relaxin, which is released in the body with the aim of making the joints and ligaments – especially in the pelvic region – more flexible in preparation for birth. Great, but the flipside is that it leaves the body vulnerable to pain and injury, back included. On top of that, there's the extra weight you're carrying around the front which affects your posture for the worse.

In most cases, pregnancy back pain will ease at some point after your baby is born. Unfortunately, you may find you're still suffering for a while as the effects of relaxin continue, often exacerbated by all the lifting and lugging you'll be doing once you've got a baby.

What can I do about it?

- Boring but true: regular, gentle exercise such as yoga, Pilates or swimming (see page 119) can help to prevent and ease backache. Strengthening your abdominal muscles is especially important, as they perform such an important role in supporting your back: try doing some pelvic tilts or 'cat' stretches daily (see page 119).

- Paying attention to your posture is vital: try to avoid standing for long periods and avoid lifting anything heavy (but, if you must, make sure you bend from the knees).

- Check the position of your computer and chair if you work at a desk.

- Ditch the high heels, as these can just make things worse.

- Try a maternity support belt, band or corset – these are made from stretchy fabric and are fixed on with straps or Velcro, with a wider panel that sits underneath the bump to give it support. You might never have considered wearing this outside of pregnancy, but may come to love it so much you're loathe to give it up once it's all over.

- Massage can help: go to a qualified professional therapist aimed at mums-to-be, or rope in your partner and get him to try some of the techniques outlined in the box below.

- If it's very bad, your doctor may prescribe pain relief medication, or refer you to a physiotherapist or other specialist.

Could it be serious?

For some women, back pain in pregnancy, especially if it's linked to pelvic girdle pain (see above), can be so severe it affects their ability to walk or move around. Let your midwife know if you're really suffering, as you can have physiotherapy.

Massage for back pain

- First find a position that's comfortable. With a bump, that's probably going to be on your side (supported with cushions if necessary), lying on a bean bag, or straddling a chair backwards.

- Ask your other half to apply gentle but firm circular strokes with the heels of his hands over the muscles of your lower back.

- Ask him to give your shoulders and neck a rub too, as tension in these areas can cause or worsen pain lower down.

- Be cautious if you're using an aromatherapy oil – some aren't suitable for pregnant women, so double-check first. If in doubt, stick with a little baby oil or olive oil.

Incontinence

What is it and why is it happening?

Inevitably, the pelvic floor muscles – which support the bladder – come under a lot of stress during pregnancy as the uterus grows. And they're more vulnerable than ever because of the release of relaxin, the hormone that loosens up a pregnant woman's muscles and ligaments in preparation for birth. So, leaking wee when you cough, laugh, sneeze or jump is a problem that affects many during pregnancy (and often afterwards as well).

'I was mortified in later pregnancy by my lack of pelvic floor control. Once I nearly completely weed myself when my husband made me laugh. Luckily we were at home when it happened and no-one else was around, but it made me feel like such an old woman.'

Claudia

What can I do about it?

Also boring but true: the single most important thing you can do to prevent or ease the problem of a leaky bladder is regular pelvic floor exercises (see page 120). Don't be tempted to try to cut out fluids, as it's important to keep well hydrated for good health.

Could it be serious?

It should get better after pregnancy – but then again, birth itself can damage the pelvic floor further and for some women this results in longer-term incontinence problems. In this case, please don't suffer in silence – talk to your GP who can refer you to a women's health physio and help you strengthen and repair any damage caused by the birth. All of which emphasises the importance of those pelvic floor exercises. Altogether now, squeeeeeze …

Indigestion and heartburn

What is it and why is it happening?

Indigestion is a pain or discomfort in the chest and upper tummy, and heartburn is a burning pain in the stomach, chest and throat – and they're both extremely common during pregnancy. Hormones cause the digestive system to relax, which leads to excess acid in the stomach. Later on, the growing womb takes up so much space that there simply isn't much room for your stomach in there. These can feature as early as the first trimester but are resoundingly common in the third.

What can I do about it?

- Try eating smaller meals, and eating slowly.

- Aim to pinpoint and cut out whichever foods are most to blame: spicy, fatty and processed foods are the usual suspects. Absolutely avoid alcohol if you're still allowing yourself the odd glass of wine – this is a big culprit for the dreaded heartburn.

- Some women say drinking a glass of cold milk helps.

- If you're particularly plagued at night, try sleeping in a propped-up position using pillows.

- Try a suitable over-the-counter antacid remedy such as Gaviscon, which gets the thumbs up from many of the *Modern Mums*. 'I developed a severe dependency on Gaviscon and would make sure that I had a supply of it with me at all times,' says Nicki, and both Claire and Beatriz confess to 'swigging it directly from the bottle'.

Could it be serious?

No, just horribly uncomfortable. And, to de-bunk a daft pregnancy myth, it doesn't mean you're going to have a hairy baby – I suffered both times, and had two baldies.

Insomnia

What is it and why is it happening?

Trouble sleeping at night can be caused by any number of other pregnancy symptoms: likely culprits are back pain, overactive bladders, heartburn and, of course, that walloping great belly that's getting in the way of you and a comfy position. And since it can also be a time of high anxiety, many pregnant women find that their nights are punctuated by strange dreams and wide-awake worrying.

On top of all that, unborn babies are often very active in the dead of night. So – as if to taunt you in advance of the many further nights of sleeplessness he intends to wreak upon you once born – your baby may be contributing to the problem with his insistence on paying homage to the karate kid in utero.

What can I do about it?

Make yourself as comfortable as possible with extra pillows – one between the legs and one under your bump can really help. Avoid caffeine after 3pm. And try to get a little exercise in the evening, or at least try some relaxation and breathing techniques (see page 170). I used to wake up at 4.38am. Every. Single. Morning. Eerily exactly the same time give or take a couple of minutes – and I couldn't get back to sleep, so I got used to listening to *Farming Today* on Radio 4 in the early hours rather than lying fretting about sleep. You may find it offers you time to do something practical and calming. I know a lot about farming now.

Could it be serious?

No, just very, very frustrating – and exhausting. But nothing like the exhaustion of being up all night with a teething baby, so it's best to break your body in gently.

Overheating and hot flushes

What is it and why is it happening?

Lots of pregnant women find the switch on their natural body thermostats goes up a notch or two, caused by the increased blood flow round the body. While a slight advantage in the winter ('I felt like I had a permanent internal central heating system – one of the bonuses of a winter baby!,' says *Modern Mum* Julie), it can add to the general misery and discomfort if you're well into pregnancy during warmer weather. And this tendency to feel the heat can sometimes come in waves, or 'hot flushes', affecting your face in particular and turning your complexion a shade of scarlet. You may find you experience some dizziness or fainting at the same time. It may also turn you into a sweaty Betty, as perspiring is the body's way of dealing with heat.

What can I do about it?

- Stick to loose clothing in natural fabrics, and wear layers so you can easily strip off if necessary.
- Keep the windows open for a bit of natural air con, and consider investing in a little electric fan if you don't have air conditioning at work.
- Don't overdo it, and don't forget to drink loads of fluids too, as you'll find your thirst levels rise with your body temperature.
- Stay indoors – and, if outside, stick to the shade.

Could it be serious?

No. Although there's evidence that a serious rise in your body temperature could be harmful to your baby, which is one reason why you're warned off saunas and very hot baths during pregnancy (see page 113 for more on that), you'd have to be very hot indeed for this to be a possibility.

Piles

What is it and why is it happening?

Ah, piles. How thoughtful of Mother Nature to scatter this particular symptom so widely and indiscriminately among the pregnant population. Medically known as haemorrhoids, these little lumpy clusters around the back passage are caused by pregnancy hormones making the veins there swell. They can be painful, itchy or both. They may bleed, and can make having a poo a wince-inducing experience (which can exacerbate the problem and cause a vicious circle if you're already suffering from constipation).

‘Up until pregnancy I thought haemorrhoids were an "old" person's problem. But no – it was quite horrifying the first time I realised I had some new friends "down there".’

Becca

What can I do about it?

- Eat lots of fibre and drink plenty of water to keep your bowel movements loose and regular.

- An ice pack or cold flannel can provide a little relief.

- You could also ask your midwife or doctor to recommend a suitable over-the-counter cream or, if they're severe, to prescribe suppositories.

Could it be serious?

No. But they're a right pain in the arse.

Rib pain

What is it and why is it happening?

Sore and tender ribs can occur, generally later on in the third trimester, as your uterus expands and pushes against the ribs. The little Mike Tyson inside you can also cause a fair amount of pain with his kicking, punching and head-butting. (Try not to take it personally … he's going to really love you when he gets out, honest.)

What can I do about it?

Stick to loose clothing, and keep an eye on your posture. A mound of well-placed cushions can aid your comfort while sitting.

Could it be serious?

No. Junior should stop using you as a punchbag once his head engages, just before birth (see page 201).

'Having twins was like hosting a party that I wasn't invited to myself. Seriously, the amount of kicking and punching going on, I'm amazed they didn't break out of my belly. The kicks in the ribs were agonising and it was hard not to shout in pain sometimes, particularly if they happened during a meeting at work.'

Rachel

Stretch marks

What is it and why is it happening?

These pink or purplish lines can appear on the belly, or anywhere else where you gain weight during pregnancy, such as your breasts or thighs, and in time they fade to become silvery. They affect some women and not others: it's all down to genetic factors that predetermine your skin type – if you're going to get them, you're going to get them.

What can I do about it?

The only really effective solutions for stretch marks will cost you a lot of money. For most women, it comes down to accepting them as an unavoidable symbol of motherhood. Massaging yourself with Bio-Oil or other oils and balms containing shea butter or rosehip seed oil will be a pleasant thing to do and may make some difference.

Could it be serious?

No, stretch marks are purely superficial. Look upon them as affectionate marks of love from your baby, a testament to how amazing your belly is that it can swell so much to accommodate your growing bub. Recently, mums started posting pictures of their post-baby bodies with stretch marks on social media after John Legend's wife Chrissy Teigen posted a photo of her stretch-marked tummy, captioned: 'You're a tiger who's earned her stripes!'

Swollen ankles, feet and fingers

What is it and why is it happening?

Swelling in the extremities is common and is caused by displaced fluids which have been forced elsewhere in the body by the increased blood flow. It can be made worse if the weather's warm, or if you've been standing for long periods.

Another reason for your feet getting bigger during pregnancy is when weight gain and softening ligaments cause your arches to drop – so your feet could easily go up a whole size or more. A bit of a nuisance if it means having to purchase new (and sensible) footwear. You could be like *Modern*

Mum Jess and embrace her love of flip-flops with an excuse to wear them for months – although make them Birkenstocks so there's some support for your feet.

‘I was totally unprepared for the fact that my feet would become like Shrek's feet! I was expecting to get a bit of swelling, but honestly! … My feet aren't swollen any more … but I gained a whole shoe size … Well … not all bad – I had an excuse to buy new shoes.’

Joanna

What can I do about it?

- Don't stand up for too long – rest and put your feet up (literally) whenever you can.

- You can help to improve blood circulation and lessen swelling by doing some simple exercises: try rotating your foot regularly, to both sides.

- A good pair of support tights can also minimise the risks – and yes, these may sound like a garment from hell, but try 'em before you knock 'em.

Could it be serious?

Generally it's harmless. But keep an eye on it and mention it to your midwife (who'll be on the alert for it in any case), as severe swelling in the hands and face can be a symptom of pre-eclampsia (see page 41).

WHEN TO GET HELP QUICKLY

Some symptoms could (although they won't necessarily) indicate a serious problem, and should be checked out as soon as possible. Get on the phone to your midwife, or make a same-day appointment with your GP, if you're experiencing one or more of the following:

- vaginal bleeding (see the box on page 66 for more on bleeding)

- severe, persistent abdominal pain

- any kind of vision disturbance

- sudden or severe swelling in the hands, face and eyes, especially if you also have a headache

- a sudden raging thirst, accompanied by a lack of urination

- very severe vomiting coupled with pain and/or fever

- fluid leaking from the vagina

- a severe headache that persists for more than a few hours

- pain or burning when you wee

- severe itching all over your body

- a lack of fetal movements after 24 weeks for high-risk pregnancies and after 28 weeks for normal pregnancies – 'count the kicks' from about 20 weeks, and if you notice a decrease in regular movement patterns, contact your midwife without delay

- frequent dizziness or fainting spells

- a heavy fall – although your baby is well cushioned inside you in his amniotic sac, it's best to be checked out after any significant knock.

If you're very concerned and you can't get hold of a medical professional, dial 999 and ask for an ambulance.

Medical factfile: bleeding in pregnancy

The appearance of any vaginal blood can be a huge worry during pregnancy, but it is common – up to one in five pregnant women experience it. Although you should always take it seriously and get advice, in most cases it will be nothing to worry about. There may not be a cause for the bleeding, but where there is, it could be one of the following.

- **Implantation bleeding:** some light bleeding, usually known as 'spotting', might appear as the embryo implants in the womb, a few days after conception.

- **Breakthrough bleeding:** spotting can sometimes occur at around the time your next period – and sometimes subsequent ones – would have been due.

- **Cervical ectropion:** this is a condition in which the cervix is affected by cell changes that make it more prone to harmless bleeding. If you bleed a little after sex, it will usually be down to this. Cervical ectropion may also be the cause of a heavy vaginal discharge.

- **A vaginal infection:** for example, vaginal thrush (see page 49) or bacterial vaginosis, which can sometimes cause a little bleeding as well as discharge; or a sexually transmitted infection such as chlamydia.

- **An underlying cause:** for example, a cervical polyp (a benign growth).

- **Placenta praevia:** this is where the placenta is low-lying in the uterus and blocks or partially blocks the cervix, from where it's more likely to detach and therefore cause bleeding, which may be severe (see also page 15).

- **Placental abruption:** a rare complication in which the placenta comes away from its implantation site. It will usually mean that an emergency caesarean section is needed and can occasionally be life-threatening to either mum or baby.

- **Spotting:** a bloody 'show' after 37 weeks could just be a sign you're close to going into labour. There's more on this on page 203.

Sadly, bleeding does occasionally signal something very serious, such as an ectopic pregnancy, a molar pregnancy, or a miscarriage. See page 28 for more on bleeding in the first trimester.

Do contact your midwife at the first sign of any sort of bleeding. It should always be taken seriously, and she will either be able to reassure you or arrange for a check-up.

YOUR BABY BUMP

Whichever of the catalogue of ailments you get lumbered with, there's one that happens to all women: a dramatic change in your body's size and shape. Most women put on between 22lbs and 28lbs during a normal pregnancy. As well as a general weight gain, which may see your face, bum and boobs (and arms and thighs, depending on your Magnum intake …) swell to a larger than normal size, there'll inevitably be a rather large protuberance in the tummy area. This will gradually push out as your baby grows, and before too long you'll be the proud owner of a lovely big, firm bump. It's the most visible sign of pregnancy and, inconvenient and uncomfortable though it can be, most women feel pretty fondly about theirs as it represents the life that's growing within.

Unwelcome touching

A word of warning: most women find that their big bellies prove a draw to all sorts of people (random strangers included), keen to stroke, poke and generally comment on it. Depending on the mood you're in, this can be one of the more irritating factors about pregnancy. Try to breathe deeply and keep smiling when you come into contact with a 'prodder'. Most mean well and are merely looking to share in the miracle of life with you – they won't realise your piles are on fire and that, frankly, you want to be stroked on the belly as much you want your eyes poked out.

If you really can't handle it, smile and take a step back. If you're feeling feisty, place your hand on the offender's belly to see how they like it.

Bumps can sometimes cause worry, as lots of women fret that theirs is too big, too small, or generally not doing what it's supposed to. It's important to remember that they come in all sorts of shapes and sizes, and they don't necessarily represent the size and shape your baby ends up either.

What your bump looks like is determined by a range of factors, including:

- the size of your baby and the placenta

- how much weight you gain

- your height and posture

- the strength of your tummy muscles (the stronger they are, the less noticeable your bump will be for a while, and the tighter it will be when it grows – hence in subsequent pregnancies you can generally expect to get fatter quicker)

- how much amniotic fluid there is

- towards the end, the position of your baby

- if you've got more than one baby in there!

It's variable, but 12 weeks is probably the earliest you'll 'start to show', as your uterus begins to push out beyond your pubic bone from here on in. Different women will start showing at different times – if you've got a good set of abs on you, or you're very slim, you're more likely to show later than someone who isn't a gym bunny or is carrying a bit of extra weight.

'I remember once being told I looked very small by one person when I got into a lift and, as I got out, someone else saying I looked like I was carrying twins! I do find it odd that the boundaries of personal communication seem to cease existing when you are pregnant. People don't tell me I look fat when I'm not pregnant, so why is it okay when I am?'

Debbie

When you have your routine checks, your midwife will probably measure your bump from top to bottom with a tape measure. If so, she's looking to check the fundal height measurement, which can give a rough idea of whether or not your baby is growing at the right rate. If you're 'small for dates' later on in pregnancy, you might be sent for a growth scan to check that all is well. Similarly, if your baby is measuring big, you may be tested for gestational diabetes.

It's all a myth that the shape and position of your bump is a clue to the gender of your baby. Inevitably, someone will tell you that if you're carrying it 'all out front' or 'low-slung', you've got a boy in there, while 'all around the sides' or 'carrying it high' indicates a girl. Humour them, but don't believe it.

STYLING YOUR BUMP

Apart from the fact that you won't see your feet for a while, and that, for a couple of months, you'll know how it feels to be a beached whale – you'll need to re-think your wardrobe.

Pregnancy and a desire to look good used to seem mutually exclusive – the words 'maternity wear' conjured up images of kaftans and baggy, unflattering clothes creating a sack-like silhouette – but that has really changed. Now we are in the era of celebrity bumps, maternity has carved out a niche fashion corner of its own. Maternity clothing has come on in leaps and bounds and there are lots of lovely, stylish brands around, and options to suit whatever your budget. Check out asos.com, Marks & Spencer and Topshop for stylish high-street options, as well as more pricey brands such as Isabella Oliver. It's important to consider how many items of maternity clothing you're actually going to need, as you're pregnant for a relatively short period in your life.

Here are a few tips.

- Be savvy with your purchases – a few key pieces can see you through your entire pregnancy and into the first months of motherhood, and end up being a worthwhile investment.

- Try undoing the buttons and zips on your own trousers and skirts – you can buy or fashion elastic loops to extend the give, if you like. Admittedly, this will take you only to a certain point in your pregnancy, but it's free.

- Once this no longer works, consider investing in a 'belly belt' or similar – a sort of stretchy fabric waistband expander that gives you more room in your normal clothes. Or you can buy maternity vests, which do the same job and are great for covering up your postnatal belly in those first few weeks after the birth. They're also great for facilitating discreet breastfeeding. More on that later.

- Dungarees are your friend – not only are they so very on trend right now, but they are comfy, stylish, bump *and* breastfeeding friendly. And, once your little one is toddling around in soft play, they are brilliant for being able to get down on the floor with them without flashing a hint of builder's bum.

- Put out a plea on Freecycle (www.freecycle.org). Someone might be looking for a new home for their old maternity wear. (It's a good place to look for other stuff that you might not want to spend loads of money on too, like your Moses basket.)

- Borrow stuff from friends who've been pregnant recently. You can always give it back if they want to extend their family later.

- Check out the maternity ranges from cheap and cheerful high street chains such as H&M, Peacocks and New Look.

- Invest in some good-quality maternity wear basics:

  ○ a pair of maternity jeans – or maybe three or four, as you can now get maternity skinny jeans, boyfriend jeans, wide-legged jeans …
  ○ a pair of smart trousers
  ○ a flattering wrap dress
  ○ a couple of tops.

The main thing to think about is the longevity of the clothes so that they work for you for a while, and remember that your style doesn't have to change just because you're pregnant. I was still wearing my maternity boyfriend jeans well into my postnatal period as they were so damn comfortable; and the maternity band is a godsend while you're still getting rid of the mum-tum. Most ranges of maternity wear include tops that work for your bump and beyond. And they're great as nursing tops – if you do choose to breastfeed, you can do so discreetly and stylishly.

Dress for comfort, above all else. Avoid anything with a tight waistband, plump for big cotton pants, don't dismiss maternity tights and leggings, and definitely ditch the stilettos.

Instagram can be a great source of inspiration for pregnancy and baby mama style. Have a look at @dresslikeamum (www.dresslikeamum.com), a mum of two from London who has made it her mission to change the way 'dressing like a mum' is perceived; she has great ideas for bump-dressing and also for breastfeeding-friendly outfits.

3 Womb with a view

Your baby's growth

HERE'S THE SCIENCE BIT

Bulls eye – you've conceived! It's pretty amazing if you stop and think about it: two people, one roll in the sack, and bingo – a baby is made. In case you're interested in the science part, here's how it happens.

- Your egg, released during ovulation, and his sperm fuse together to become one cell, known as the zygote (not to be confused with an enemy race from *Star Trek*).

- This then divides to form a cluster of cells, which travels down the fallopian tube to your uterus (womb).

- Two or three days later, implantation occurs – in other words, the fertilised egg settles down into your womb's lining.

- At this point it becomes an embryo, and, technically speaking, you're preggers – but it will be another fortnight before you're likely to suspect it, or you can take a test that will let you know for sure.

And so begins a nine-month journey of astonishing growth as your baby's life rapidly begins to unfold. Each pregnancy is unique and yours may progress slightly differently from the next woman's. Babies' weight and length measurements can vary a whole lot, too. But the following gives a rough guide to what's going on inside you during those nine magical months.

Talking in weeks

Although often described as a nine-month-long experience, medical folk measure the progress of pregnancy in weeks, since the changes you go through are so rapid, and it's important that specific tabs are kept on your progress. It might sound a bit faffy now, but you'll soon find yourself ticking off the time in weeks and trimesters.

HOW YOUR BABY GROWS, FORTNIGHT BY FORTNIGHT

First trimester

Pregnancy is officially dated from the first day of your last period – in other words, two weeks prior to conception. So you're already two weeks 'pregnant' before you've actually got pregnant, and by week six, the life inside you has only really been there for four weeks Confused? You will be.

At six weeks

- The tiny embryo in your uterus, safely encased in a little bag called the amniotic sac, is just 4–6mm in size.

- His neural tube – which will eventually become the brain and spine – has already started to develop, his vital organs are in place and his heart has begun to beat.

- He has little 'buds' where his limbs will soon be emerging, an emerging head, and dimples which will become his ears.

The placenta

Part of the cluster of cells that implanted will now develop into the placenta – the organ that links your blood supply to the baby's, and

---

through which oxygen and nutrients are passed from you to your baby, via the umbilical cord. The same system carries waste from the baby out again. The placenta also helps protect your baby from infection as it passes on antibodies from you, and produces hormones that will sustain his growth and development in the womb.

At eight weeks

- Your baby is no longer an embryo, but a prawn-shaped fetus (the word means 'young one') and he's around 1–2cm long.

- Although he's bobbing around in amniotic fluid – the colourless liquid that's helping to protect him in the womb – you won't feel his movements for a while yet, although they could be detected from now by ultrasound scan.

- His face is slowly forming too, and he has small dark splodges where his eyes will be. His skin is transparent and paper-thin.

'I was surprised by how much I felt like a mum straight away, worrying about this little bean from the offing (and still now!) despite never being a worrier before.'

Julie

At 10 weeks

- Your baby is now around 2–4cm long (this is known as the crown to rump length – in other words, what he measures from head to bottom).

- He has a disproportionately large head, but his body is beginning to straighten.

- His facial features – including the beginnings of the nose and upper lip – and limbs continue to grow.

'I had had a couple of miscarriages and so this pregnancy was quite a stressful one to begin with. Just before my scan, at around 10 weeks, I had a really vivid dream where I heard my baby's heartbeat and could see him soft and warm inside. It was so strong that I just knew everything was going to be okay. And it was.'

Rowan

At 12 weeks

- He's now fully formed. His skeleton is complete and all his body parts are in place, including the sex organs.

- He can suck, swallow and yawn.

- He continues to be active, but you still won't feel it yet.

- His fingers and toes have separated and his hair is growing – though the colour of it could well change after he's born.

- His eyes are fully formed but still closed, and his sense of hearing is developing.

- He already has the beginnings of his teeth – even though they won't usually make an appearance until he's five or six months old.

One trimester down ...

Getting to week 13 is a real turning point in pregnancy, because you're through the risky first trimester, when most miscarriages occur, and your chances of losing the baby become very small. It's usual to have a dating scan around now, giving you an exciting and reassuring glimpse of the bun that's in your oven.

Second trimester

At 14 weeks

- Your baby's length is approximately 8–10cm.

- He has a recognisable chin, forehead and nose.

- He'll start to develop a fine covering of downy body hair, known as lanugo – which is probably there to keep him warm until he's laid down sufficient body fat to do so.

- He's already in possession of his own unique set of fingerprints.

Heartbeats

From now on, your midwife may use a Doppler – a handheld ultrasound machine – to locate and listen to your baby's heartbeat. A normal fetal heart rate (FHR) can be anywhere between 110bpm and 160bpm, but on average it will be around 140–150 beats per minute – twice as fast as a normal adult's.

At 16 weeks

- He can wave his fingers, toes and limbs around now.

- He has little fingernails in place, and may be able to suck his thumb.

- His ears are developing and he can hear your voice, as well as your heartbeat and the rumblings and grumblings of your digestive system.

'I first felt my baby definitely at 16 weeks. It felt like little bubbles, little punches biffing me gently inside. When I had the scan his little fists were punching me in exactly the way I had imagined!'

Manna

First movements

You may just about be able to make out your baby's movement from now on. At first it feels like a fluttering or bubbling sensation – it's very

> easily confused with a bout of indigestion and so is often overlooked for quite a while in a first pregnancy. Don't worry if you can't feel anything yet – it's still early days, and you should pick up on your baby's movements some time in the next four to six weeks.

At 18 weeks

- He's 13–15cm in length now.

- He can punch, kick, turn and wriggle and he may be passing the time in there by tugging and swinging on his own umbilical cord.

- His head is still large in comparison to his body, but his face is becoming more and more human in appearance. He's also pulling a range of faces.

- Although his eyes are still shut, they'll be sensitive to bright lights from outside.

- He's begun to practise his breathing skills in preparation for his exit, by inhaling and exhaling amniotic fluid.

'I had been feeling my baby for a few weeks, tentatively at first and then definitely. But the most amazing time was when my boyfriend first put his hand on my belly and felt movement for himself. I think he was quite overwhelmed by it.'

Jess

At 20 weeks

- He's beginning to get a waxy coating known as vernix to protect his skin from the soaking it's getting – most will be gone by the time he's born, but there may well be traces left.

- His hearing is well developed and he may jump or jerk at loud noises.

- His taste buds are developing.

- He'll be growing eyelashes and eyebrows.

Halfway point

You're halfway there, and you should be offered an anomaly scan now or very soon. It's usually possible for the sonographer to tell whether or not your little one is in possession of a willy (fairly accurately – but it's not guaranteed). However, you might have to ask for this information – and some hospitals still have a policy of not letting on at all.

At 22 weeks

- Your baby's crown to rump measurement will be somewhere around 18–20cm now.

- His head and body size will have evened out so he's in proportion – a small but perfectly formed version of the fully cooked baby you'll get to meet later on.

- He can hear and recognise your voice, so you might want to talk or sing to him – he'll find it soothing and may even give you a small kick or elbow of acknowledgement for your troubles.

'I used to lie on my bed and spend ages looking at my belly moving. It was amazing. Absolutely the best part of being pregnant for me was being able to feel my baby kicking and squirming around inside.'

Maria

At 24 weeks

- His lungs are strengthening and he'll be practising his breathing by inhaling and exhaling amniotic fluid. This sometimes causes him to have hiccups, which you can feel.

- His skin will still be wrinkly, as he's yet to fill out to his birth weight.

- He has fully formed eyes.

'I learnt more about my husband through my pregnancy. I am a reader and a sharer. He is not. So all the "I'm growing eyebrows inside my belly" comments were kind of lost on him. We grew closer in a lot of ways and I learnt that he is a lot harder to scare than I am.'

Kat

Viability

From this week, your baby is considered to be viable, which means that he'd stand a chance of survival in a neonatal intensive care unit if he were born now.

At 26 weeks

- He'll open his eyes for the first time around now.

- You'll probably be well aware of all his somersaults, kicks and karate chops – unfortunately, babies in the womb often like to do most of their partying at night.

'I became aware of sounds that she reacted to: transport noise, sudden loud noises, music (like the 'Mad Men' theme tune that she heard a lot!). It was amazing feeling her personality developing inside.'

Manna

Third trimester

At 28 weeks

- His brain continues to develop and it's thought that around this time babies may begin to dream – about what, no-one knows!

- Visual responses are up and running – if you were to shine a torch at your belly, he'd turn his head to find out who put the lights on.

- His transparent skin is beginning to turn opaque.

'I loved the third trimester – it was when I really bonded with the person inside me. You instinctively rub your belly and acknowledge the baby as they move inside you. You get to know when they like to sleep and be active. When they have hiccups and are having a stretch. You'll never be as physically close to that baby again. Once they are born you can feel a little helpless in keeping them well and safe.'

Debbie

The home stretch

Phew – you're in your third and final trimester. Your baby's really starting to fill out your uterus and, as it gets more and more crowded in there, you're likely to feel more and more uncomfortable. The reassuring news is that your baby's chances of survival, should he be born prematurely, are now very good indeed.

At 30 weeks

- Your baby should now be around 28cm long, and weigh an average 3lbs.
- His wrinkly skin will be smoothing out as he gets plumper.
- His lungs and digestive tract are almost fully formed.

Movement worries

You may find your baby becomes less active than he has been. It's nothing to worry about, it's just that there's less room in there for his aqua-aerobics sessions.

Lots of mums feel anxiety when their babies slow down or stop moving altogether for a while, especially if they've been hyper beforehand.

However, it's very normal for movement to be erratic and you probably won't need to panic. It's really important to notice and get to know your baby's own pattern, so you're more likely to realise if it changes.

If you haven't felt a normal amount of movement from your baby during the period when he's usually most active, try sitting quietly for a while and drinking a glass of iced water or a sugary drink – as your bladder fills up with chilly liquid, it should provoke some movement. If it doesn't, and you're still concerned, let your midwife know.

‘Sometimes I would freak out if I suddenly thought I hadn't felt him for a while. I'd have a glass of coke or a cold glass of water, and push him a bit to see if I could wake him up. Thankfully, usually he'd kick in annoyance for me disturbing his nap! It was always a relief.’

Sophie

At 32 weeks

- He may be lying head down in preparation for birth by now, but there's still loads of time for him to turn.

- His sleeping cycles may be longer, so he may be quieter for longer periods.

- The lanugo (hair) covering his body will now begin to fall out.

Positioning is everything

Your midwife will keep an eye on your baby's position by feeling your abdomen during your routine checks: if your baby doesn't get into pole position as you get closer to D-day, your obstetrician may carry out an external cephalic version (ECV) to avoid a breech birth. There are also tricks you can try to encourage him to turn round (see page 200).

At 34 weeks

- Your baby now measures somewhere around 32cm in length, and weighs about 5lbs.

- He can open and close his eyelids and focus on his own fingers.

- Most of his organs are now fully mature, except for his lungs, which still have a bit more developing to do.

- He's built up some fat deposits under his skin.

It's crowded in there

There's not a lot of room left in your uterus now and you may be getting prodded and poked a great deal, which can be surprisingly painful – you may find yourself cursing your little passenger.

However, it's endlessly entertaining when you can feel or see an elbow or foot protruding from your belly, alien-style, or when you watch as his movements cause ripples across the surface of your tummy.

At 36 weeks

- His brain and nervous system are now fully developed and his bones are beginning to harden – although the skull remains soft and flexible (hence the soft spot that your baby will have for up to 18 months after his birth) so that he can make it through the birth canal.

- If your baby is a boy, his testicles will normally have begun their descent from the abdomen into the scrotum.

- His lungs are now almost fully developed and in a week's time he'll be officially full-term. If born, he's unlikely to have any major problems and may not even need any special care.

'At around 37 weeks I started to feel like baby was really low down in my pelvis, so low I worried she might actually drop out while I was walking around Tesco!'

Natalie

Breech babies

Most babies will have moved into the 'head-first' position by now but a small number remain stubbornly in the 'breech' (bottom-down) position, or even sideways (see page 200) – and some move round only to flip back again a bit later. You may soon feel pressure low in your abdomen, caused by the 'engagement' or 'lightening' process, as the baby drops down in preparation for birth. Some babies don't engage until the last minute, though.

At 38 weeks

- He's likely to be around 6–7lbs in weight now and is definitely full-term (term starts at 37 weeks).

- He'll have lost most or all of his hairy, waxy coatings. He has swallowed them and will poo them out again after he's born!

- He won't be moving so vigorously – he just doesn't have the room!

'At 38 weeks my baby was so strong it really felt she was trying to push her way out. My husband used to love just laying his hands on my bump and playing karate with the little one and you could really see her shape – hands, arms, knees – pressing through my skin. He couldn't believe how strong she was. Neither could I! My poor organs were being bashed around inside.'

Ruth

On guard

It's time to be on your guard for signs of labour – there's a more detailed guide to these on page 203.

At 40 weeks

- He's an average 35–37cm from crown to rump.

- He weighs anything from 6lbs to 8lbs on average.

- He's got fully developed internal organs.

- He's definitely ripe and ready now. If you haven't yet gone into labour, you soon will!

Is that it?

Some pregnancies go on for 42 or even 43 weeks. Your midwife will keep a very close eye on you from now on – sometimes labour may need a helping hand (see page 204).

4 Care instructions

Eating, drinking, and other potentially 'dangerous' activities

ADAPT YOUR LIFE, DON'T DITCH IT!

Eat this, avoid that, squeeze these: it's crazy the amount of instruction you're given in pregnancy when it comes to your health and that of your baby – the list of what you should and shouldn't eat, drink, inhale or otherwise subject your body to seems to go on forever. If you followed every one of the guidelines to the letter, you'd be carrying around a list of rules and regulations as big as your bump.

It's true that they're all there with the best of intentions: to warn you of any potential risk (however minuscule) for your baby. Unfortunately, official guidance tends to skirt vaguely around the subject without any useful pointers as to precisely what the consequences might be, or how likely they actually are. So you end up having to choose between erring on the side of caution (and feeling neurotic and deprived), or throwing caution to the wind (and feeling rebellious, anxious and guilty).

I played it fairly safe with my first baby, and was very careful not to eat and drink things that were on the 'Don't' list. I then had a couple of miscarriages after having him, and although I had stuck to the 'rules' to the letter, I inevitably agonised about various things I might have done, imbibed or ingested to 'cause' them. My second baby was my fifth pregnancy, so I had been through the anxious first trimester quite a few times, and this last time I felt a slightly more fatalistic sense that I shouldn't change my 'normal' way of being. This, of course, is with the understanding that I wasn't exactly a crazy hedonist in the first place (I did have a toddler, so, let's face it, I wasn't out dancing on tables every night), but I do like a glass of red. So I carried on having a regular glass of wine every weekend night, eating runny eggs, doing yoga … and I didn't fret about them. Both my babies, when they finally arrived, were perfect, thankfully – but yes, if anything had happened, I would probably have regretted every single little risk item I ever consumed, on the off-chance that it was something I could have avoided.

I can't tell you whether to be rigid or relaxed about the pregnancy rulebook. What I can do is guide you through all the official advice, which, as you can see from the real-life opinions I've included, is advice that not everyone chooses to take. Maybe you will decide to take the rules with a pinch of salt, or maybe you'll want to follow them to the letter, just to be sure. Do whatever makes this pregnancy work best for you.

The bottom line is this: we're talking guidelines here, not laws. And, ultimately, the lifestyle you keep during pregnancy is down to you.

ALCOHOL

Can I have a drink during pregnancy or not?

I'm going to be bad cop here, but in general you should be thinking about the absolute minimal alcohol intake during your pregnancy, and certainly never get drunk once you know that you're pregnant (unknowing benders in the past? – let bygones be bygones). In 2008, NICE and NHS guidelines were revised to say that pregnant women were given the official thumbs up to indulge in one or two drinks a couple of times a week. These guidelines were reviewed in 2014, remained unchanged, and have now been moved to a 'static' list, which means they will stay as such for the foreseeable.

The official guidelines from the NHS are: 'Women who are pregnant or trying to conceive should avoid alcohol altogether. However, if they do choose to drink, to minimise the risk to the baby, we recommend they should not drink more than one or two units once or twice a week and should not get drunk.' The 'however' caveat is unhelpfully slightly wishy-washy and leaves the onus on you to decide what to do for the best for you and baby. If in any doubt, and if it's likely to cause you to worry (not good for baby in itself), just leave the prosecco off your shopping list for the next nine months or so. And maybe try to convince your partner to give up with you in solidarity, as him continuing as normal can make abstaining feel even harder. But if you know that having one small glass of an evening, once or twice a week, will be a pleasure you simply can't forgo, continue without fretting about it. Make sure you don't drink on an empty stomach, as the liver can process alcohol more efficiently if you've eaten.

'"Holy shit! We are fucking pregnant." My first thought was that I was gutted that I couldn't drink the bottle of delicious red wine that we had bought for dinner.'

Jenn

'I kept my pregnancy hidden but I was feeling really rough. I didn't take any time off, but backed off from the social side of things – my boss guessed in the end when I wasn't drinking at the Christmas party.'

Bella

The truth is that doctors still aren't completely sure how much alcohol is safe to drink in pregnancy. But they do know that women are drinking more heavily in general these days, that measures are bigger, and that many drinks are stronger. So one 'glass' of wine can mean lots of different things in terms of how much alcohol you're actually consuming. The NICE guidelines suggest that you abstain altogether in the crucial first trimester. For some, that ship has sailed if you find out you're pregnant after a particularly hedonistic weekend. But you might feel 'safest' giving up the sauce completely once you know you're pregnant, for that short period of time at least, for peace of mind.

Alcohol passes from a woman's bloodstream into her baby's through the placenta, and excessive drinking is definitely potentially harmful. Babies born to women who drink heavily during pregnancy – in other words, anyone downing more than six units a day, which can be just two large glasses in one sitting, depending on the size of the glass – are at significant risk of being born with a condition called fetal alcohol syndrome, which can cause facial deformities, restricted growth, and learning and behavioural difficulties. It will also increase your risk of:

- having a miscarriage (during the first trimester)
- your baby's organs, nervous system and growth being affected
- premature birth, or a low birth weight (which means your baby is more vulnerable to infections and other health problems)
- your baby being more susceptible to illness later in life
- suffering a stillbirth.

On the face of it, this new advice is pretty bad news for women who find it hard to face the possibility of 40 entirely dry weeks.

Fortunately, however, all the official bodies go on to point out that there is no evidence that *light* drinking during pregnancy is harmful, and say that, for women who do choose to drink, a 'safe amount' is one or two units, no more than once or twice a week.

'I found out I was pregnant two days before my honeymoon, which meant that my one and only all-inclusive experience had to be limited to mocktails.'

Julia

'I treated myself to a glass of wine every single night of my pregnancy and decided not to worry about it. I wasn't out getting leathered, I was simply savouring one delicious glass. In my mind there was absolutely nothing wrong with that.'

Kate

What's a unit?

Wine	Units at ABV 12%	Units at ABV 14%
Small (125ml) glass of wine	1.5	1.75
Standard (175ml) glass of wine	2.1	2.45
Large (250ml) glass of wine	3	3.5

Drink	Units
330ml bottle of 5% strength lager	1.7
Pint of 5% strength lager	2.8
25ml measure of spirits	1
35ml measure of spirits (usual amount served in pubs)	1.4
Double (50ml) measure of spirits	2
275ml bottle of alcopop (ABV 5%)	1.4

Remember that some wines will have a higher than average ABV content, which can push the unit total up a little further. If you want to know more, there's lots of information, plus a handy online units calculator, on the website of the Drinkaware Trust.

On the safe side

So the main points to remember about enjoying a tipple or two in pregnancy, are as follows.

- You don't have to give up booze altogether. If you want to stick to the recommended 'safe levels' of alcohol during pregnancy, aim for a maximum of one to two units a week, drunk just once, or twice, per week. Some experts still suggest you should forgo booze altogether in the first trimester, though.

- When drinking, don't forget that measures these days are generous and alcohol content may be higher than you realise, so count your units and the alcohol by volume (ABV) content of your glass (see the tables above).

- Don't 'binge' drink – in other words, don't consume more than six units in one session (and I appreciate that may be stating the bleedin' obvious, but I mention it just in case you were thinking of getting totally rat-arsed while knowingly pregnant ...). That said, you shouldn't worry if you were drunk on the odd occasion before you knew you were up the duff: you're unlikely to have caused any harm as it's prolonged heavy drinking that's most risky.

CIGARETTES

Should I give up smoking when I'm pregnant?

In a word, yes. If you smoke while pregnant, your risk of miscarriage and stillbirth increases by 26%; you're more likely to suffer some kind of complication such as placental abruption (see page 67); and there's more chance of your baby having a low birth weight (according to NHS statistics, babies of mothers who smoke are, on average, about 7oz lighter at birth than others) or being born premature, and therefore more likely to suffer infections or other health problems. Once born, your baby is more likely to have poor lung function and to suffer from difficulties in feeding and breathing (asthma, for instance), or chest and ear infections. Smoking is also one of the established risk factors for cot death – so it makes absolute sense for you both to stop now, before you've got a baby in the house.

Does it matter that I smoked before I knew?

There's no need to worry if you smoked before you knew you were pregnant – you won't have harmed your baby in doing so because the risks outlined above are linked to pregnancies where mums have smoked throughout. As long as you stop at some point in your first trimester, your baby will be fine. If you really can't stop, you should certainly aim to smoke as little as possible. There are places you can go to ask for help with quitting smoking – ask your GP or in your local Boots.

Quit while you're ahead

Pregnancy is the best excuse you'll ever have to kick the habit, and for good. Lots of women find it's a natural point at which to cut out smoking – and they don't even miss it much. So, if morning sickness or just general good intentions provide you with the motivation to give up, make the most of it. And if your partner smokes, urge him to quit too: not only will it provide you with support, it will mean your home becomes smoke-free, and that's going to be so much better for your baby once born.

There's lots of advice about giving up smoking available on the NHS website Smoke Free or by calling the NHS pregnancy smoking helpline (see page 273). Nicotine replacement therapy is free on prescription in pregnancy, but should only be used after appropriate advice and an assessment from a health professional such as your GP or local stop smoking service specialist adviser. The sooner you can stop, the better for you and your baby.

‘I'd been meaning to give up smoking for ages and not quite committing to it. Becoming pregnant was the push I needed, as my conscience couldn't deal with putting my unborn baby at risk. So I stopped as soon as I found out, and haven't looked back.’

Maria

DRUGS

Regular medication

If you take regular medication for a chronic or long-term condition such as diabetes, asthma or epilepsy, make your doctor aware of your pregnancy straightaway (that's if you haven't already sought their advice while trying to conceive). Don't stop taking your drugs without getting medical advice first, though.

Over-the-counter stuff

Pregnant women are generally advised to avoid over-the-counter medication unless it's really essential. However, you're fine to take the odd recommended dose of paracetamol, and certain essential remedies like Gaviscon, which tackles heartburn, are okay. If in doubt, ask your midwife, GP or the pharmacist before taking or applying anything, or give NHS 111 a call. And don't assume that alternative or herbal remedies will be okay because they're 'natural' – some also have risks. Again, check with your midwife first.

Illegal drugs

Apart from the obvious risks to your own physical and mental health, taking any sort of illegal recreational drug during pregnancy could certainly be harmful to your baby. While research in the area is somewhat sketchy, it's known that regular use of cannabis increases the risk of low birth weight and slow growth; speed increases the risk of congenital deformities; and ecstasy pushes up the risk of birth abnormalities. Cocaine is particularly dangerous stuff during pregnancy as it can trigger miscarriage, early labour or placental abruption (see page 67), and it may cause brain damage, disabilities or even death in an unborn baby.

If you did take illegal drugs on a one-off or occasional basis before you knew you were pregnant, it's unlikely to have caused your baby harm, but it's important to come clean with your doctor or midwife so they can make sure you have any additional antenatal checks that might be needed. If you have an actual drug addiction, it's vital you get it sorted out, so you'll need to tell your midwife or GP about it. They won't (or shouldn't) judge you for it.

CAFFEINE

Your daily brew

You'd think after all that abstinence you could at least put the kettle on and enjoy a limitless stream of your favourite hot beverage, wouldn't you? Sadly not.

The advice of the Food Standards Agency (FSA), the government's independent authority on food and nutrition, is that 200mg of caffeine is the safe daily limit to aim for in pregnancy.

That's just two mugs of instant coffee or one and a half of a decent brew – and, of course, caffeine can also be found in tea, cola and other soft drinks, chocolate, and certain medicines – see the list below. Reassuringly, the FSA points out that if you occasionally have more than this you shouldn't worry, as 'the risks are likely to be very small'.

Fortunately for many women, nature has its own way of overturning entrenched caffeine habits (and this goes for the booze and fags, too): if you're suffering from morning sickness, the tea and coffee you previously loved may now seem about as appetising as a bowl of cold vomit.

Why is it risky?

It's thought that high levels of caffeine can increase the risk of low birth weight, making a baby more vulnerable to a range of health problems, and there's some evidence that links a very high consumption to miscarriage. Excessive amounts may also trigger or worsen a range of general health problems such as insomnia, headaches, increased blood pressure and dehydration – all of which you could well do without when pregnant.

How much caffeine does it contain?

- Mug of instant coffee: 100mg

- Mug of fresh brewed or filter coffee: 140mg

- Mug of tea: 75mg

- Can of cola: 33mg

- Can of energy drink: 80mg

- 50g bar of plain chocolate: 50mg

- 50g bar of milk chocolate: 25mg

- Two-capsule dose of max strength cold and flu remedy: 50mg

'I've always drunk a lot of coffee but suddenly when pregnant I was craving more and more, up to eight cups a day at work. It was really hard to cut down. I switched to decaf but it didn't taste as good.'

Berit

FOOD

Was it something I ate?

There are certain bugs that, if passed on to an unborn baby, could have a harmful effect on them. In pregnancy, your immune system is weakened, which means you're slightly more at risk of picking up infections than usual but, even so, the chances of your baby contracting any of the infections outlined below and being harmed as a result are small. (And in some cases they're minute.)

If you *do* suspect you've contracted anything potentially harmful, you should contact your GP at the earliest opportunity, since speedy treatment can prevent the infection reaching your baby.

Raw or undercooked meat

Undercooked or raw meat can harbour the toxoplasma parasite, which can cause an illness called toxoplasmosis. Most of us have already had it and are immune to it, and in a healthy adult it usually causes nothing more than mild, usually flu-like symptoms. But in a very small number of cases (around 800 babies a year are infected, with 10% of those affected as a result), it can lead to serious illness or birth defects in an unborn child, miscarriage or stillbirth.

'When I found out I was pregnant I panicked initially, not about the coming nine months, but about the next few days! I had just placed my order for our work Christmas lunch – rare steak – and was wondering how I could dodge all the scrutiny of not drinking and whether I could get away with changing my meal order without telling anyone.'

Manna

- If you want to avoid the risk altogether, you should ensure your meat is well cooked, particularly poultry and minced meat products like sausages and burgers. No rare steaks or pink burgers on the BBQ.
- Heat anything that comes from a packet until it's steaming hot all the way through.
- Pay careful attention to food hygiene where raw meat storage and preparation are concerned (see also page 104).
- It's also recommended that you avoid raw meats such as salami, pastrami and Parma ham – although these are all fine if cooked, for instance when they're on top of a pizza.

Unwashed fruit, veg and salad

Soil may also harbour toxoplasma, so official advice is to wash fruit, veg and salad well before eating. Some experts recommend that you do so even with the packaged, pre-washed varieties, just to be on the safe side.

Mould-ripened or blue-veined cheeses

It's advised that you forgo cheeses such as stilton, brie, camembert, roquefort and dolcelatte in pregnancy because they may contain listeria, a bacterium that can cause an infection called listeriosis. It's incredibly rare (infection occurs in one in 30,000 pregnancies, with the chance of harm to your baby even smaller still) but, although it may result in nothing more than mild, flu-like symptoms in a pregnant woman, it can lead to serious illnesses such as meningitis, pneumonia, jaundice, premature birth or even death in an unborn baby.

'I was pregnant over Christmas. A glass of port with stilton and crackers is my favourite thing. I was gutted to have to skip it but I couldn't face the worry if I indulged.'

Rowan

As well as avoiding the high-risk foods, you can avoid catching the listeria bug by being scrupulous about food hygiene (see the box below).

Pregnancy food myth busted!

You don't have to give up blue or squidgy cheeses completely if you don't want to. Cooking them through will remove the (already pretty small) risk of listeria, so there's nothing wrong with a bit of stilton soup or some deep-fried brie if you're hankering for a whiffy fix. You don't have to avoid all soft cheeses, either, only those that are mould-ripened or made with unpasteurised milk. So ricotta, mozzarella, mascarpone, cottage cheese and cream cheese are all absolutely fine.

Raw or undercooked eggs

Undercooked eggs (and poultry) may, just rarely, contain salmonella, a bacterium that causes a very nasty form of food poisoning with symptoms that include vomiting, diarrhoea, severe head and stomach pain and fever. While particularly unpleasant to go through in pregnancy, it's very unlikely to cause any harm to your baby, although it can lead to dehydration, which can cause complications. So if you've suffered a nasty bout, seek advice from your midwife or doctor.

To play it safe, make sure you cook eggs through before eating. And don't despair if you can't bear eggs boiled till they bounce – as long as they're lightly cooked they're fine (see below). More of a risk is anything that contains uncooked or partially cooked eggs: home-made versions of mayonnaise, hollandaise sauce, ice cream, and certain fresh puds such as chocolate mousse, for instance – so if you're dining out, or with friends, you might want to ask first. The pre-packaged shop-bought varieties of these things are fine because they'll have been made with pasteurised eggs (in other words, heated to a point that would destroy any bacteria).

'I kept eating "bad" things by accident, like Parma ham or runny eggs. Then I'd find out they were on the "don't" list and worry. But nothing bad happened, so I think I'll be more relaxed next time.'

Kirsty

Pregnancy food myth busted!

You don't have to avoid runny or lightly cooked eggs. As long as the whites are no longer translucent, they're cooked enough to be safe. You'll also (almost certainly) be OK if you stick with the 'lion-stamped' eggs as these are inoculated against salmonella. You don't have to avoid mayonnaise, either – as long as it comes out of a jar, it's fine. (And really, does anyone actually make their own?)

Machine ice cream

Soft ice cream that comes out of a machine is best avoided in pregnancy because it's kept at a lower temperature and there's always the risk the machine will be harbouring bacteria. Bad news if you have a penchant for Mr Whippy. Stick with ice cream from a tub, if you want to be certain.

Liver

It's thought that an extremely high intake of the retinol (animal) form of vitamin A can cause birth abnormalities – so since liver (and liver products such as liver pâté and liver sausage) contains fairly large amounts of the stuff, the official advice is to avoid it altogether. However, as you'd need to have a pretty serious liver habit for it to be risky, you've no need to worry if you had some before you knew you were pregnant. Cod liver oil supplements also contain the retinol form of vitamin A, but not in any quantity that could be dangerous – so again, don't panic if you were taking these before you knew you were pregnant.

'I went to a wedding in France in my first trimester … when I was trying to keep my pregnancy secret. I was surrounded by delicious wine, amazing smelly cheeses, foie gras, and not wanting to eat them but knowing if I didn't everyone would guess why. It was a nightmare.'

Faye

Raw (unpasteurised) milk or cheeses

These are known to sometimes harbour bacteria such as those that cause listeria, toxoplasmosis and salmonella (see above), so you're advised to avoid them in pregnancy. Virtually all the milk and milk products you'll find in the supermarket are pasteurised, and unpasteurised milk is generally only available from specialist suppliers (it's also known as 'green top'), so it's easy enough to avoid. Goat's and sheep's milk, and their products, are often unpasteurised, so if you rely on them because of an allergy or intolerance to cow's milk, you should double-check.

> ## Pregnancy food myth busted!
>
> Probiotic yoghurts, drinks and other products are all perfectly safe. They do contain bacteria, but only the 'friendly' sort, which are good for us. Sour cream is fine, too.

Shellfish

It's considered sensible to avoid raw or undercooked shellfish such as prawns, mussels and oysters, as they can harbour bacteria that cause food poisoning such as salmonella (see above) and campylobacter, another very common germ. As a general rule, shellfish won't cause you any grief if you cook them before eating, or have them as part of a hot meal, but they're probably best avoided from buffets where they may have been hanging around; from fish counters or stalls where you're not sure of the quality; or in ready-prepared sandwiches from sources you don't entirely trust (you really ought to be fine if you get them from a reputable purveyor of prawn sarnies such as M&S – that's your call, though).

> ## Pregnancy food myth busted!
>
> You don't have to avoid prawns altogether. They're absolutely fine if heated completely through (so stir fries and curries are okay) and you can also eat them cold as long as they're very fresh, they came pre-packaged and dated (rather than loose), and you eat them the same day.

Raw fish

Advice varies on whether or not you should give up smoked salmon, trout and mackerel during pregnancy (as it's been smoked, rather than cooked, it's partially raw). The FSA says the risk is negligible, and, if you're wobbling on this one, bear in mind that you'll almost certainly be fine if you stick to the stuff that comes pre-packaged and dated, and refrigerate and eat it quickly. The NHS guidelines are that smoked fish is totally fine to eat – always stick to the general rules of food hygiene and preparation and you should be good to go with your smoked salmon and cream cheese bagel.

Sushi gets the go-ahead in general, as it's usually been frozen beforehand, which will kill any parasites that might be hanging around. You'll be okay if you buy it from a supermarket or make it at home (freezing it first, for 24 hours), but if you're in a restaurant where the fish is likely to be fresh and possibly unfrozen, ask first to check.

'I used to live in Japan and sashimi is one of my favourite treats. I avoided it completely until I realised that Japanese women probably eat fresh raw fish and are fine, so I continued to have it occasionally.'

Nainna

Oily fish

Although generally a very nutritious food as it contains omega oils that can help prevent heart disease and may boost the development of an unborn baby's nervous system, it's advised that you limit your consumption of oily fish such as fresh tuna (canned tuna doesn't count as 'oily'), mackerel, salmon, sardines and trout during pregnancy as they've been fund to contain pollutants. FSA guidelines recommend no more than two portions a week.

Fish with a high mercury content

Fish that may contain mercury, which can damage a baby's nervous system, are also best avoided: shark, swordfish and marlin. Tuna is absolutely fine to eat in limited amounts: the FSA suggests no more than two fresh steaks or four cans of the stuff weekly.

Fresh pâté

As a fresh product that can hang around on shelves for a while but doesn't go through a heating process before consumption, pâté comes with a (tiny) risk of listeria – official advice warns against meat, fish and even vegetable varieties, although you'll be fine with those that come in a tin or are vacuum-packed. Liver pâté is a no-no anyway, because of the risks of too much vitamin A (see liver, above).

Peanuts and peanut products

Official advice on this is non-committal, as research into the matter is ongoing and authorities including the FSA and the NHS want to wait for more evidence before issuing a whole new set of guidelines. At the time of writing, both bodies say that if you're pregnant and in a high-risk group (in other words, if you or your baby's dad has an allergy or an allergic condition such as eczema), you 'might want to' steer clear of peanuts and peanut products. If that's you, chat to your GP or midwife about it and do some careful research before making any decisions. We've included some sources of further information on food safety at the back of the book.

Pregnancy food myth busted!

Eating peanuts won't give your baby a peanut allergy. The jury's still out, but in fact some doctors are beginning to suspect that, if anything, early exposure to allergens may be beneficial.

You certainly don't need to avoid nuts if there is no history of allergy or an allergic condition in your immediate family.

Barbecues and buffets

Bacteria breed quickly on food that's left uncovered in a warm place, so you might prefer to stick to food that's come fresh off the barbie, and be selective when it comes to party spreads, steering clear of stuff such as open jars of mayonnaise, prawns or cold meats, for example.

Chilled, unwrapped deli foods, restaurant food and takeaways

By 'deli' foods, I mean things like cold meats, quiches, pies and salads. In the strictest terms, you'd give all these things up, because you just can't be certain of their hygiene history, but it would hardly be realistic. You *ought* to be fine with cold food from a reputable shop or establishment. But if you're still not convinced, the main thing to bear in mind is that anything's OK if it's been (freshly) cooked or thoroughly heated through.

Diet food and drinks, and artificial sweeteners

There has been much hoo-ha in the press over the years about the potential evils of artificial sweeteners such as aspartame, and it means that you're unlikely to be able to bring a can of Diet Coke to your lips while pregnant without some hesitation or worries about disapproving glances. So, here are the facts: artificial sweeteners are just that – artificial. Therefore they are human-created chemical concoctions rather than naturally occurring sugars. The diet industry has utilised them over the past half a century to reduce the amount of sugar used without losing the sweet taste, therefore lowering the number of calories a food contains. And if you believe all the claims made against them you would assume they were responsible for all sorts of potentially harmful conditions such as cancer, strokes, seizures, low birth weight, high blood pressure ... the list goes on. Aspartame has a particularly bad rep, being linked to brain tumours. Studies conducted by the European Food Safety Authority in 2013 confirmed that there is little evidence of a link between consuming aspartame and an increased risk of developing cancer, and have determined that pregnant women and children are perfectly safe to continue consuming aspartame and other sweeteners. The NHS website concludes that, as part of a healthy balanced diet (that's the key here, ladies), sweeteners have a really important role to play in allowing you to enjoy as much of a sweet taste as you desire while staying within healthy calorie limits. Time for a Diet Coke break ...?

STAYING ZEN

It's hardly surprising that so many women end up getting quite stressed over what they're supposed to avoid in pregnancy – the list goes on forever, the risks in some cases seem so minute, and advice seems to differ depending on what you're reading or who you're talking to.

Whatever you do, try not to worry too much about food safety. Play it 100% safe if it feels the right thing to do, but don't let it become a source of high anxiety. Because that's something that *definitely* isn't good for you, or your baby.

A HEALTHY APPROACH

Why eat well?

Time for another boring-but-truism: it makes sense to eat as healthily as possible during pregnancy. If you're eating well you'll boost your immune system and have all the energy you need to meet the extra physical demands you're under. You'll also be less likely to pile on too many excess unwanted pounds. And a good diet will also help boost the growth and development of your baby in a number of ways. Certainly, it's a good idea to steer clear of a *really* crap diet if you can: one recent study found that babies born to mums who ate lots of junk food are more likely to suffer health problems such as heart disease and diabetes later in their own lives.

Tips for good food hygiene

- Keep your kitchen clean.
- Wash your hands thoroughly before and after handling food.
- Thoroughly wash all fruit and veg.

- Defrost frozen meat and other foods thoroughly, preferably in the fridge.
- Cover food when in the fridge, and store raw and cooked products separately.
- Make sure all hot food is served piping.
- Make sure your fridge and freezer are the correct temperatures (0°C to 4°C for fridges, below 18°C for freezers).
- Chill or freeze food as soon as you get it home from the shop.
- Have separate chopping boards for raw foods and foods that are ready to eat.
- Eat food within the use-by dates.
- Keep pets out of the kitchen.

Okay, so eating a healthy diet in pregnancy is easier said than done. For many of us, morning sickness in the first trimester (and sometimes beyond) puts paid to a nutritious intake – or any intake at all, in some cases. I survived on a daily diet of toast and Ribena – the only two items I could stomach – for a period of about two months in my first pregnancy. Other women have far-from-nutritious food cravings that simply have to be indulged. And then, of course, there's the fact that pregnancy is a time of so few guilty pleasures. Booze, cigs and rare meat are off limits. So, if you can't turn to cake, crisps and chocolate in a bid to cheer yourself up, what else is there?

Beware of 'eating for two'

It's normal and natural to gain weight and for your shape to change during pregnancy: you are never, ever going to have such a brilliant excuse for the pounds piling on, and you will never have a better reason for a stomach that sticks out. After all, you're growing an extra person in there, not to mention housing a ruddy great placenta and the natural resources in your breasts for keeping the baby nourished after her birth.

However, it's worth bearing in mind that the 'eating for two' excuse is a bit of a myth – I realise this is going to make me unpopular, but I have to report that the demands of pregnancy can be met with an average increase of no more than 200–300 calories a day, and that's only in the final trimester. Shame, that. Quite apart from the extra work involved in losing your baby bulges a bit later down the line, putting on too much weight can put you at higher risk of developing conditions such as pre-eclampsia (see page 41) and gestational diabetes (see below), as well as putting extra strain on your body in general and making difficulties during birth and labour more of a likelihood. And the truth is that a lot of women do put on more weight than is healthy for them in pregnancy.

So, tempting though it is to keep your spirits up by gorging on chocolate and cake, don't go overboard. There's no need to be obsessive – just aim for a broadly healthy diet with a good variation of different foods.

'Thinking about it, I loved how I looked when I had a proper bump. I was really proud of it. I expected to mourn the loss of my pre-pregnancy body but, actually, I loved my new shape!'

Natalie

How much weight should I gain?

It varies hugely depending on the size you started out at, but the average woman can normally expect to put on anywhere between 22lbs and 28lbs. Only a third of that is accounted for by your baby – the rest is a combination of extra breast tissue, your growing uterus, the placenta, amniotic fluid, increased blood volume, extra fluid and fat stores.

The guidelines published by NICE, the National Institute for Health and Care Excellence, in 2010 (due to be reviewed in July 2016) focus on your being a healthy weight and BMI throughout pregnancy rather than indicating a specific figure in terms of pounds gained. You are pregnant, and the key is to stay at a healthy weight rather than fret too much about the escalating number on the scales. And it will escalate, which for some of us is quite a hard concept to embrace at first, particularly if you're used to being 'in control' when it comes to your shape and weight.

As long as you're not living purely on chocolate and cake, your weight gain is likely to be absolutely 'normal', as we all lay fat down differently in pregnancy just as we do in normal life – during my first pregnancy I seemed to put on all my weight on my arms, back and face (annoying), but my bottom half remained slim. *Modern Mum* Faye laments that everything she ate plastered itself immediately onto her bottom and thighs. There's an element of relaxing yourself into your growing new shape, while trying to stay as healthy and active as you comfortably can throughout the trimesters. No-one is ever going to deny a heavily pregnant woman ice cream, though.

'The best thing about being pregnant was finally loving my body and being amazed at what it was doing. It was the first time that I have enjoyed growing larger, as it meant things were progressing as they should.'

Nicki

In the US, they have a very general rule of thumb based on the one-two-three principle.

- If you were overweight before you got pregnant, you should expect to gain no more than one stone.
- If you were a normal weight before you got pregnant, you should aim to gain around two stone.
- If you were underweight, you should aim to gain about three stone.

Medical factfile: gestational diabetes

Being overweight or gaining lots of weight are risk factors for a pregnancy-related condition called gestational diabetes. Gestational diabetes is also more common if a parent or sibling has diabetes, if you are over 30 years old or of Afro-Caribbean or Asian descent.

Diabetes occurs when the body doesn't make enough of the hormone insulin or doesn't respond to it so well, causing high levels of blood sugar. In pregnancy you need to make more insulin for the sake of your baby as you become more resistant to its action, and for a small number of women, the body can't achieve this extra demand.

With gestational diabetes, you risk ending up with a bigger than expected baby and therefore a more complicated birth, with caesarean section more likely. It could also cause your baby health problems after his birth. Healthy eating and exercise are usually enough to keep blood sugar levels under control, but sometimes treatment in the form of tablets or insulin injections is needed.

If in doubt, don't worry

It may be reassuring to remember that the female body is a miracle vessel that can foster new life in spite of adversity – as demonstrated by the fact that Third World mothers close to starvation can gestate, give birth to and even feed their babies.

Do try to eat as healthily as you can, but *don't* beat yourself up if you're not consuming the perfect balance of foods you know you're supposed to. *My Pregnancy Recipes and Meal Planner* (White Ladder, 2014) includes lots of pregnancy-friendly recipes, and helps you plan what you eat – to satiate cravings but still get the nutrients you and your baby need.

What to aim for in a healthy pregnancy diet

- **Fruit and veg:** Five portions a day is the minimum recommended. Remember that you can include lots of things that don't really feel like fruit and veg at all: baked beans, tomato-based pasta sauces and fruit smoothies, for example. I'm not sure if carrot cake is accepted though …

- **Starchy foods (carbs):** Aim for three or four servings of bread, rice, pasta or cereals a day, and plump for the healthier wholegrain or brown varieties whenever possible, which will help to ease constipation.

- **Protein:** Get at least two servings a day, in the form of meat, fish, eggs, beans or pulses.

- **Eat three meals a day:** But also well-timed snacks to keep you going in between. Nutritious nibbles include fresh and dried fruit, yoghurts and cheese, wholemeal bread or toast, or a bowl of non-sugary cereal.

- **Calcium:** Really important for the growth and development of your baby's teeth and bones – however, you don't need any more in pregnancy than the RDA (recommended daily allowance) for an ordinary adult female, which is 700mg a day. That's a daily glass of milk (230mg), a pot of yoghurt (225mg) and a matchbox-sized piece of hard cheese (288mg).

Alternative sources of calcium

- Canned sardines (430mg per can)
- Bread (83mg per two slices of white or wholemeal)
- Baked beans (100mg per small can)
- Nuts such as almonds (30mg per six nuts)
- Green vegetables such as broccoli (35mg per two florets)

Some products are fortified with extra calcium – certain cereals, orange juice, soya and tofu, for example – so it's always worth checking the labels.

- **Vitamin D:** This ensures your baby's bones develop well and also boosts the content in your breast milk, which is already in production. Food sources include fortified margarines, eggs, meat and oily fish, but it's mostly provided by the sunlight we're exposed to (it's sometimes called 'the sunshine vitamin'). Some women are more vulnerable to vitamin D deficiency than others – those with dark skin, those who cover their skin, don't get out in the sunlight much, or don't get enough foods that are rich in vitamin D. The government recommends that all pregnant women take a 10 microgram (mcg) supplement of vitamin D daily.

- **Iron:** Requirements rise in pregnancy, because you're keeping your baby well supplied with it, too. Good sources of iron are red meat, leafy green vegetables (spinach, watercress and broccoli, for instance), shellfish, eggs, dried fruits such as apricots or figs, nuts, pulses and beans, whole-meal bread, fortified breakfast cereals and dark chocolate. Your doctor or midwife may suggest iron tablets if they're worried that you're seriously lacking it, but with some caution as they can cause constipation – already a prominent pregnancy side effect for many women. There's more information about iron-deficiency anaemia on page 30.

- **Folic acid:** Taken prior to conception and during the first trimester, it can help to protect against neural tube defects such as spina bifida, a condition which can cause serious disabilities. You can get a certain amount from foods such as leafy green veg (spinach, sprouts or greens), citrus fruits and fortified breakfast cereals. However, official advice is to take a 400mcg supplement of the stuff daily until your 12th week of pregnancy. Folic acid supplement tablets are readily available in chemists and supermarkets, and it's also included in most antenatal multivitamin supplements.

- **Omega 3 (or essential) fatty acids:** This is rumoured to help boost your baby's brain and eyesight development, but there's little evidence to support this theory. Oily fish is the best source – mackerel, sardines, kippers, salmon and fresh tuna. (Canned tuna won't cut it, as most of the healthy oils are removed in the canning process. However, tinned varieties of other oily fish, such as mackerel, sardines and herrings, are okay.) If you don't like or don't eat fish, you can get a certain amount of omega 3 from nuts and seeds such as pumpkin and sunflower seeds, and from the fatty king of the fruit, avocado.

- **Drink lots:** Water's the healthiest drink around, but you can also get your daily fluid intakes from tea and coffee (of course, there's the recommended caffeine limits to take into account), fruit juices (very high in sugars, remember – so limit them, drink with meals, and dilute with water where possible), and milk (which will boost your calcium intake, too).

Pregnancy isn't the time to be on a weight-loss diet, so any calorie-counting or carb-avoiding should definitely be ditched. If you're worried about gaining more weight than you'd wish to, simply concentrate on a broadly healthy diet, as outlined above, and keep active (see the section on exercise later in this chapter).

If your diet is seriously restricted, perhaps because you're a vegan, or for a medical or religious reason, let your GP or midwife know. They may recommend a supplement, or refer you to a dietician for some extra advice.

Should I take an antenatal supplement?

The best way to get most of the nutrients we need is through the food we eat – and that means anyone who has a normal balanced diet will be fine. However, the current recommendation of the Department of Health is that all pregnant women take 400mcg of folic acid, for the first 12 weeks, and 10mcg of vitamin D, throughout pregnancy (and during breastfeeding, too). You can buy these separately from most chemists and supermarkets, or try and get hold of the Healthy Start vitamins, which the government provides to pregnant women on benefits, and which contain the recommended amounts of folic acid and vitamin D, as well as some vitamin C. In some areas, you might be able to buy these very cheaply through your primary care trust (some experts think they should be routinely available to all women anyway). It's worth asking your midwife, just in case.

You really don't need a general pregnancy multivitamin. Antenatal supplements can be pricey, and they contain lots of things that you probably don't particularly need. If you decide to take one, stick to supermarket or chemist own brands, which are always cheaper.

If you're taking a mix of supplements, make sure you're not taking more than the recommended daily allowance of anything, as too much could be harmful for your baby.

OTHER 'DANGEROUS' ACTIVITIES

Apart from the mass of information regarding what to eat and drink, what else should be avoided in pregnancy? As with food, it's basically down to you. But here are some of the activities where a possible risk (in some cases, a very small one) has been identified.

Beauty and spa treatments

Colouring your hair

This a subject that generates lots of debate, but there's no real evidence that colouring your hair will harm your baby. Some tests have suggested it may be harmful if absorbed through the scalp and into the bloodstream, but these involved huge quantities of the chemicals in question. So, the good news for those among us who would rather spend nine months in a cupboard than let the world see our roots is that colouring your hair in pregnancy is almost certainly safe.

It's worth bearing in mind, though, that hormonal changes affect your hair's condition so you might get a different colour or texture from the one you bargained on. You're also more likely to suffer an allergic reaction than usual, so do a strand test first.

If you're really worried and prefer to err on the side of caution, you might choose to avoid colouring your hair during the first trimester when the baby's early development takes place, as some experts recommend. Or you could stick with streaks or highlights, which aren't applied right up to the roots and so can't be absorbed into the scalp, or vegetable-based dyes. When you do dye, take the usual sensible precautions and be sure to wear gloves and apply it in a well-ventilated area. Of course, if you're suffering from morning sickness, you may find the smell of the fumes is an even worse prospect than your roots beginning to show.

Fake tan and sunbeds

Some experts say it's advisable not to use fake tan during pregnancy, because you're more at risk of allergic reactions – you should be fine as long as you do a patch test first. Although most fake tans are safe to use during pregnancy, there are some that you might consider avoiding.

The active ingredients in fake tan work by interacting with the skin cells in the top layer of your skin. When they're rubbed onto your skin as a mousse or cream, they aren't absorbed into the bloodstream. But if you use a spray or a spray-tanning booth, chances are you might inhale some of the active ingredients, and it's not known how breathing in fake tan spray could affect you or your baby.

Just to be on the safe side, try to avoid tanning booths for the duration of your pregnancy, and stick to fake tans that you can apply by rubbing. If you absolutely can't live without your regular brand and do want to use a spray at home, make sure the room is well ventilated.

Trying to get a sunbed tan isn't a great idea either – partly because some research links increased UV rays with folic acid deficiency, and partly because hormone levels can affect skin pigmentation, which means you may suffer from chloasma if you use a sunbed (or, indeed, if you sunbathe).

Saunas, hot tubs, steam baths and Jacuzzis

Getting so hot that your body temperature rises isn't recommended, partly because it may push up the rate of your baby's heartbeat, and partly because it can affect blood pressure and cause fainting or dizziness. There's also some evidence of a link between very serious overheating and damage to your baby's nervous system.

For the same reasons, pregnant women are traditionally advised to avoid extremely hot baths and to take care not to overdo it while exercising. So hot tubs and other such indulgences are probably best avoided, and if you're fond of a deep, hot soak, aim to keep your bath water a comfortable temperature – not so hot it turns your skin pink.

Aromatherapy

This is a great way to aid relaxation and help other pregnancy niggles, but some essential oils are believed to be unsuitable, and even potentially risky during pregnancy. Your best bet is to stick with treatment from a qualified practitioner who is registered with the Aromatherapy Council.

At home

Gardening

Because soil can contain the toxoplasmosis bug (see page 96), there's a tiny risk of infection if you get it on your hands. You'll be fine if you wear gardening gloves and wash your hands thoroughly when you're done.

Exposure to paints

Water-based household paints (like emulsions) won't have a harmful effect on your baby. However, the NHS points out that little research has been carried out on the matter and suggests that, although if there *is* a risk it's a very small one, you should avoid painting in the first trimester.

Solvent-based paints, varnishes and brush cleaners are more likely to cause harm than water-based ones, so it's recommended you don't get creative with these. It's also a good idea to avoid stripping any old paintwork, since, way back before the 1970s, paint sometimes contained elements of lead, which can be poisonous.

Household chemicals and cleaning products

This is another area where there's no firm evidence of danger either way. However, it makes sense to avoid powerful products such as pesticides and oven cleaners just to be on the safe side – and, let's face it, who wants to be doing cleaning when they're pregnant anyway?

Contact with animals

Cat poo can harbour toxoplasmosis, so don't empty litter trays if you can help it, and use rubber gloves if you must. Bacteria is found in animal waste generally, so it's sensible to wash your hands after contact with pets.

Out and about

Air travel

There's no reason at all why you can't fly during an uncomplicated pregnancy, other than the fact that it may make you feel more wretched during the first trimester if you're suffering from morning sickness, and that if, later on in pregnancy, you happen to go into labour it's a bit awkward to say the least. (If you've had any issues with blood pressure or bleeding, or if you have a medical condition such as diabetes, do check with your doctor first.) Some airlines get twitchy about pregnant travellers from 28 weeks, and may refuse to take you or insist on a doctor's note confirming you're fit to fly. (Policies vary, so always check before booking.) The risk of DVT (see page 37) increases when you're pregnant, so you're well advised to move around a lot during any flight, and consider wearing support stockings – low on glamour, but high on practicality.

The main thing to bear in mind about going away is that, depending on where you are going, you need to be happy that you can access good care for yourself and your baby at your destination, and are happy to stay overseas if you happen to deliver prematurely. You should also check the small print in your insurance policy, to make sure it covers pregnancy and care for a newborn baby if the unexpected happens.

Mountaineering, skiing and hot air ballooning

I'm all for carrying on as normal, but common sense has to dictate that some activities are simply not suitable when you're pregnant. Your sense of balance is affected while pregnant so anything that relies on that is probably worth giving a miss to be safe, and anything that might cause you to fall and knock your bump is probably best avoided. Official advice is to avoid these pastimes since the high altitudes involved mean a change in oxygen levels, and that could potentially trigger a miscarriage. Scuba-diving is also considered a no-no during pregnancy because of some evidence that it could put an unborn baby at risk of decompression sickness (better known as the bends) and cause an increased risk of miscarriage.

Theme park rides

Rapid stops and starts can damage the womb and are thus best avoided. Water slides should probably be enjoyed with caution – most pools display a warning notice to steer clear if you're expecting.

At work

Using computers

There's no evidence of any risk to your baby as a result of regular computer use, which is a shame because it would be a darn good excuse to get signed off an office job for the duration. There's more on specific risks at work in the following chapter.

And finally … x-rays

In most cases the risk from diagnostic x-rays is low and, if you absolutely have to have one for some reason, it doesn't mean your baby will be harmed. However, doctors are likely to advise you to wait until after your baby is born if the x-ray isn't urgent. If your dentist needs to carry out a mouth x-ray, he'll provide a protective apron to wear over your belly.

> ## Infections that could harm your baby
>
> Some contagious infections could be harmful for your baby if you're affected by them during pregnancy, including rubella, chicken pox and parvovirus B19 (slapped cheek syndrome). It's pretty unlikely you'll pick one of these up because most of us have immunity already, but if someone you've been in contact with has one and you suspect or are worried that you might have caught it, do let your midwife or GP know, so they can take tests where necessary and do whatever they can to treat you and your baby.

DON'T STOP MOVING

It might be a bitter pill to swallow if you've never been a fan of exercise, but pregnancy isn't a time to stop moving altogether. In fact, if you're not already used to it, starting up gentle exercise when you become pregnant is a great way of managing the various aches, pains and gripes of pregnancy and making you feel a whole lot better in body and spirit.

As well as boosting your general fitness, flexibility and health, exercise can aid relaxation, reduce aches and pains, improve sleep, offset constipation, and help prepare you for the physical demands of late pregnancy, labour and birth, and for caring for a new baby. Research suggests that if you keep fit during pregnancy, you're more likely to have a shorter labour time and fewer delivery complications. It may also reduce the risk of developing certain pregnancy complications.

If you were a couch potato before pregnancy, now isn't the time to take up a strenuous new regime, so aim for something fairly gentle such as walking, swimming, or organised sessions specifically designed for pregnancy, such as aqua-natal classes or antenatal yoga.

If you were already fit, you can keep up the same level of activity as before for as long as you feel comfortable doing so. But bear in mind that, while it's okay to try to maintain your fitness, you definitely don't want to be training to improve it – at least, not unless you're Paula Radcliffe (and even she had to slow down a bit when expecting her daughter).

Fortunately, your body's unlikely to allow you to overdo it, so listen to what it's saying – if you're knackered, slow down or stop, and if you experience any specific problem such as bleeding or dizziness (see the full list on page 122), get some professional advice before continuing. If you've always been a bit of a gym bunny, or you like to pound the pavement, you may have to accept that four or more major sessions a week are just too much right now and bring things down a notch. Or you may be like *Modern Mum* Nicki and compete in a triathlon at 14 weeks pregnant ... it's all relative to what your own body is used to, but I wouldn't recommend *beginning* triathlon training for the first time ever while pregnant.

'I think I did too much, thought pregnant women were whingers. However, doing body pump until 34 weeks took its toll and I used to wake up with terrible cramp in my calves.'

Melissa

The risk of injury can be reduced by making sure you do warm-up and cool-down exercises either side of a workout. A decent pair of trainers, where trainers are required, is also important.

Whatever your level of fitness, you'd be wise to fit in at least a little every-day activity where possible, and, if nothing else, keep up your pelvic floor exercises. Your bladder will thank you if you do (and so will your man, it's said). There's more about pelvic floor exercises on page 120.

What sort of exercise is suitable?

Some regular aerobic (cardiovascular) exercise – the sort that raises your heart rate, such as power-walking, running, dancing and low-impact aerobic classes – is fine during pregnancy if it's what your body is used to. If you never did that kind of exercise before, or if your body's asking you politely to take it down a notch, stick to walking at an ordinary (but brisk) pace or swimming to give your heart and muscles a gentle workout.

Swimming in particular is a much-recommended way to exercise in pregnancy as the buoyancy of the water will support you and your bump and it is low impact, and therefore unlikely to leave you injured. However, the leg action of breaststroke can put pressure on the lower back and pelvis, particularly if you tend to swim with your head out of the water, so stick to front or back crawl if you're suffering from pain in those areas.

If getting sweaty or wet isn't your sort of thing, you may prefer to concentrate on strength conditioning exercises such as yoga or Pilates. These can improve your muscle tone and flexibility, but won't improve your cardiovascular fitness (ideally, you'd do a bit of both sorts of exercise). They're especially good in pregnancy, as they can help to strengthen the 'core' muscles of your pelvic floor and lower abdomen, and they're particularly relaxing ways of exercising. Look for a class designed for antenatal requirements, because there are certain positions and postures that aren't suitable when you're pregnant. Check out the website of the Guild of Pregnancy and Postnatal Exercise Instructors to find your nearest qualified instructor.

If you fancy doing some gentle strength conditioning exercises at home, try some daily pelvic tilts.

- Stand with your shoulders and bottom against a wall, keeping your knees soft.
- Tilt your pelvis, so that your back flattens against the wall, and hold for about four seconds, continuing to breathe.
- Repeat up to 10 times.

Or try 'the cat'.

- Get down on all fours with your hands below your shoulders and gently hold in your tummy, so that your back is flat.

- Now draw in your tummy and tilt your pelvis so that your bottom tucks under and your back rounds upwards and your head curls underneath.

- Hold for a few seconds, return to the neutral position, then repeat.

Squeezy-peasy: the importance of pelvic floor exercises

Your pelvic floor is a layer of muscles that form a supportive 'hammock' for your bladder, bowel and uterus and, inevitably, it comes in for a massive hit while supporting a growing baby for nine months (and then playing a key role in its expulsion at the end of it all). As a result, many women who've been through pregnancy and childbirth develop a tendency to leak urine when coughing, sneezing, exercising or laughing.

Pelvic floor exercises (sometimes called Kegels after the obstetrician who pioneered the idea) carried out regularly through pregnancy and after birth can make a real difference in preventing this. And if that's not enough incentive for you, try this: they'll help increase sensitivity during sex and strengthen your orgasms.

The good news is that they're not difficult and you can do them any time, any place – at your desk, waiting at traffic lights, watching telly, while washing up, etc. – and no-one will be any the wiser. Here's how:

- First, identify where your pelvic floor muscles are. The best way to do this is to imagine you're trying to stop breaking wind, and then imagine stopping the flow of wee mid-flow (don't ever try this when you are actually weeing). This engagement from the front to the back of the pelvis will find the full expanse of the pelvic floor. Check you're not tensing your tummy, buttock or thighs, as these aren't the muscles you're looking for – it's a purely inward engagement, nothing externally should grip or change.

- Try squeezing and releasing the muscles quickly, repeating up to 10 times.

- Then squeeze slowly, trying to hold the muscles tight for up to 10 seconds before relaxing. Repeat this 10 times.

- Ideally, you should do both sets of squeezes four to six times a day. And remember: the 'release' part is just as important for when you're actually giving birth.

- A useful tip is to put little coloured stickers in various places throughout your home and in the car, as reminders to do a few squeezes when you see them. Nobody else needs to know what they're for.

Take the stairs

Plenty of women lack time, energy or motivation to do any formal exercise when pregnant. And if you're someone who hates working out at the best of times, you're hardly likely to become a convert while feeling sick, heavy or tired. But, if nothing else, aim at least to fit some sort of activity into your life so you don't really notice it – take the stairs instead of the lift, and walk whenever you possibly can.

Can exercise be risky?

The main risk in exercising during pregnancy is injuring yourself. However, there's also a very small possibility that, if your body temperature shoots through the roof during the first trimester, it could damage your baby's developing nervous system. It's pretty unlikely you could work out so hard you make yourself this hot – and the body thermostat is set at a lower level than normal in pregnancy, providing a natural safety mechanism. But still, it's a good idea to drink plenty of water before, during and after exercise; to wear appropriate clothing; not to work out in very hot and humid weather; and to avoid overexerting yourself.

Use the 'talk test' to give a good indication of how your body's coping: you should be able to continue a conversation while exercising without catching your breath.

Any extreme sports are also out of bounds – for obvious safety reasons.

What about my netball/riding/hockey/rugby?

If you've always participated keenly in a regular sporting activity of some kind, you may wonder if and when you should stop when you're pregnant. You'll probably know yourself how risky something feels, and how much a big, round stomach is likely to affect your balance and general prowess – so it's basically down to you whether you carry on. However, the experts tend to suggest that you should give up any type of sport that poses a significant risk of back and other injuries (weight training, rowing, tennis), losing your balance and falling (gymnastics, ice hockey, skiing, cycling, horse-riding), or being inadvertently walloped (kickboxing, judo, football, rugby). You may find that once you've got a baby inside you, your keenness for these kinds of things will waver in any case.

When you shouldn't exercise

Exercise may not be a good idea if you have a chronic condition or if your pregnancy is affected by any sort of complication – if one develops, you might have to stop. If in any doubt, check with your doctor or midwife. Generally speaking, you should stop exercising and seek prompt advice if you experience one or more of the following symptoms:

- dizziness or feeling faint
- headache
- shortness of breath on exertion/exercising
- pain or palpitations in your chest

- pain in your abdomen, back or pubic area, or in your pelvic girdle
- weakness in your muscles
- pain or swelling in your leg(s)
- painful uterine contractions
- fewer movements from your baby
- leakage of your amniotic fluid
- vaginal bleeding.

5 Office politics

Pregnancy and your career

YOUR RIGHTS AND RESPONSIBILITIES

For a lot of us, pregnancy coincides with a time in your life where you're sailing with a good wind in your career and fully in control of where your working life is headed, and it can be very strange and scary contemplating the idea of taking a break from what may have utterly dominated your daily life for the past decade. Or, you might be delighted about the upcoming hiatus and looking forward to a holiday from it – tip: it's a common misconception that when you're on maternity leave you're on holiday. I can vouch for the fact that many women find that *work* feels like the holiday once you've been in charge of a chaotic, messy, utterly-dependent-every-hour-of-the-day baby for a few months. It's important to be fully informed of what your employment rights are, and what you might expect over the next few months. Also, you'll find tips on how you can maintain momentum with your career and hit the ground running rather than stumbling if and when you choose to go back to work post-baby.

‘Work were fine, more or less. I was pregnant around the same time as a close colleague and it was shocking the comments we received about being a pregnancy tag team. People seemed to think it was okay just to make any random personal comments.’

Debbie

124

'The funniest thing is trying to field questions from younger colleagues who are still burning the candle at both ends and who find even the prospect of being pregnant fairly repulsive. They feign interest – and are the ones most likely to say "Wow, how BIG you are becoming." They also ask if you are looking forward to a year "OFF" – ha ha!! – and whether you are planning to come back to work after the baby (perhaps they can wheedle a promotion out of this news).'

Becca

However important your career is to you, being pregnant can really take the shine off your working day. Of course, it's not an ideal world – but there are choices to be made. In most cases maternity leave won't begin until a month or so before your due date, if not later, and until then you must simply plough on at work while doing your best to tackle the full range of physical and mental disadvantages that pregnancy can wreak.

You might also feel a bit wobbly about your impending maternity leave, wondering who's going to keep things running smoothly in your role while you're gone – or worse, that the person who does take over turns out to be better at it than you are. Maybe you're having to kiss goodbye to that promotion you've been working towards – or even fear this could be the end of your career entirely. These are all very understandable concerns – in discussions with the *Modern Mums* for this book, work concerns ranked most highly among the postnatal fears. Let's face it, up until now men haven't had to ever face a similar career break, usually at a point when you're riding the crest of a wave in terms of building your skills and experience, not to mention your earnings.

The attitude of your boss and your colleagues will inevitably affect how you cope with your career during pregnancy. If we all lived in that ideal world, every pregnant woman would have the respect, support and sympathy of her manager and fellow workers – but sadly, for some, the reality is rather different.

When to tell your boss the news

You don't have to tell your boss that you're pregnant for quite a while, if you don't want to – but you must do so before you're 25 weeks pregnant. In fact, it's sensible to let them know as early as you can, so that any necessary plans can be put in place and your risk assessment (see below) can be carried out. If you're not ready for the rest of your colleagues to know, you can always ask your boss to keep schtum for a while. But chances are you'll be rumbled early on by some bright spark who's picked up on the fact that you're permanently green around the gills, have virtually set up camp in the toilet, and are no longer the first person standing at the bar come Friday evening.

'Work were really supportive and I was congratulated. I didn't feel sidelined. I think it helped me working in the civil service. I'm sure it would have been more difficult if I was in the private sector.'

Ele

When you do come clean, you need to let your boss know what date your baby is due and when you want your maternity leave and pay to start (see below). You might be required to do this in writing. You'll also need to present them with your maternity certificate (form MAT B1), which your midwife will give to you after you're 21 weeks pregnant and which confirms your due date. Your employer must then give you written confirmation of your return date within 28 days – and unless you tell them otherwise, they must assume you're going to take your full maternity leave entitlement of 12 months. You *can* tell your boss if you know for sure that you want to come back before the full entitlement period is up (don't worry – it won't be set in stone – you can change your mind if you want, as long as you give eight weeks' notice of your revised return date).

Many women choose to wait and see how they feel, anyway. Once you've spent some time with your baby you may find you enjoy it so much you want to be at home for longer than you'd originally planned. Then again, you might realise what an easy life you had before and be champing at the bit to get back to it. Or you may just have done some sums and realised that, financially, you don't have much choice.

'They were all very positive to my face, but there were a few comments, like from my MD – "How the hell did that happen?" I wanted to be treated the same and I was … I had lots of responsibility and I made it very clear that nothing changes and they can just buzz off – and I guess they knew me well enough to know that I meant it.'

Joanna

Legal rights

What follows is only a basic guide to your legal rights as a pregnant employee. It's a complex subject and one woman's entitlements can differ from another's, depending on a variety of factors. If you've got a helpful human resources manager or well-informed boss who's prepared to take the matter out of your hands, you're in luck. Otherwise, though, you may need to do your homework to make sure your entitlements are being met.

MATERNITY LEAVE AND PAY

All pregnant employees have the right to take up to 12 months off work – it doesn't matter how long you've worked for a company, or what your hours are. The first 26 weeks of maternity leave are called Ordinary Maternity Leave (OML). You can begin OML up to 11 weeks before your baby is due – the medical view is that eight weeks is a sensible time to take off before your due date, although most women prefer to waddle into work for as long as humanly possible, giving them more time off with their baby once he's born.

If you decide on a leaving date and then change your mind for some reason, you're required to give 28 days' notice (although some bosses may be prepared to be more flexible about that). If you have to take time off work because of medical issues related to your pregnancy in the four weeks before your due date, you're automatically considered to have begun your OML. And if you give birth before your planned leave kicks off, your maternity leave will be considered to have started from then.

You should still be entitled to any contractual benefits you might get (gym membership, for example) during your leave, and your company must continue to make contributions to your pension if they do that already. You're also entitled to take any holiday that builds up in your maternity period – lots of women choose to use this to boost their total amount of maternity leave.

If you were working for an employer when you became pregnant, and you're earning more than £112 a week, you qualify for statutory maternity pay (SMP). This is paid through your employer and (at the time of writing) is 90% of your average pay for the first six weeks, and then £139.58 per week (or 90% of your average earnings if that's less) for a further 33 weeks. Note: if you decide to take the full year's maternity leave, the last three months of leave will be unpaid.

Some companies have their own maternity pay schemes in place, and you may find that your employer will offer you a more generous rate of maternity pay than the statutory rate. However, this often depends on your having worked there for a certain length of time and is usually on the basis that you'll return to work for a certain period when your maternity leave is over. If you decide not to go back to work because you want to stay at home with your baby, you may have to pay some maternity pay back.

You may not be entitled to get SMP, for instance if you started your job after becoming pregnant, or if you're a casual worker, self-employed, unemployed or on a low wage. In these cases, you can usually claim Maternity Allowance instead, which is currently £139.58 per week for 39 weeks, or 90% of your average pay, whichever is the smaller. This is paid by the government, and you'll need a claim form (MA1) – you can download this from the Department for Work and Pensions website.

If you're not sure about what you're entitled to and how to get it, the best source of basic information is the GOV.UK website.

'Whilst I was on maternity leave, I applied for a promotion and was sifted out on very flimsy criteria, and then there was a restructure and I had no say in which role I was posted to. I work for a flexible and inclusive employer, but even there, it's clear that there is a long way to go to achieve real equality for working parents.'

Bella

YOUR PARTNER'S PATERNITY RIGHTS

In April 2015, new rules came into force regarding the sharing of parental leave between the two parents. The new rules replace 'additional paternity leave', which allowed maternity leave to be divided between both parents, and the father could take up to 26 weeks' leave to care for the child if the mother went back to work 20 weeks after the birth. Now, eligible parents can take leave at different times or double up by taking leave at the same time, for up to 50 weeks, 37 of which will be paid. Mothers must still take the first two weeks after the birth of their child, but can then exchange traditional maternity leave for shared parental leave.

Both parents have a flexible choice about how to split their 50 weeks of leave – they can take it in one continuous block or in smaller chunks of time. For example, the mother could decide to take off 10 weeks after the birth, and then she and her partner would be able to choose how to split the remaining 40 weeks of leave. She could choose to take another 30 weeks and her partner take 10, or they could both take 20 weeks at different or at coinciding times.

The difference from the old rules is that the leave does not have to be taken all in one go, even if only the mother chooses to use shared parental leave rather than taking up traditional maternity leave. A parent can book up to three blocks of leave during the child's first year, and they have to give their employer eight weeks' notice of each block. A mother can also let her employer know before her baby is born that she doesn't plan to use all of her 52 weeks' maternity leave and wants to convert some of it into shared parental leave. Her partner could then use his share in the first few weeks after birth, so both parents are on leave at the same time.

To take shared leave, one parent must have been an employee with at least 26 weeks of service with the same employer by the end of the 15th week before the baby is due. The other parent must have worked for at least 26 weeks in the 66 weeks leading up to the due date and have earned at least £30 a week in 13 of those 66 weeks. Self-employed parents, and a parent not in work at the time of the birth, can still qualify.

Pay for shared parental leave is currently £139.58 a week (this will change slightly each financial year), or 90% of an employee's average weekly earnings, whichever is lower. This is virtually the same as statutory maternity pay – the only difference is that, during the first six weeks, SMP amounts to 90% of whatever the employee earns, with no maximum. Some employers may offer an enhanced package but there is no legal requirement for them to do so.

Shared parental pay is given for only 37 weeks. The remaining 13 weeks of leave entitlement, if taken, is unpaid. Go to www.gov.uk/shared-parental-leave-and-pay for more information.

TIME OFF FOR ANTENATAL CARE

Your employer must let you have time off for anything that counts as an antenatal care appointment – and this could even include something like a relaxation or parentcraft class if your midwife or GP has advised you to attend them. If your employer is the suspicious type, they might demand to see an appointment card or a note from a health professional.

YOUR HEALTH AND SAFETY

By law, your employer must do whatever it takes to protect your health and safety during pregnancy, because if they fail to do so it's automatically considered sex discrimination. Once you've formally notified your employer that you're pregnant, in writing, they must carry out a specific risk assessment based on your individual needs. If any risks are identified you must be informed, and your employer must let you know what they will do to make sure you're not exposed to them. You should make sure they know about any medical advice you've been given by a GP or midwife, ideally backed up with a note. Obviously, it depends on what your job is, but some potential workplace risks are:

- standing or sitting for long periods of time

- work-related stress

- workstations and posture

- long working hours

- mental and physical fatigue

- lifting or carrying heavy loads

- threat of violence

- exposure to infectious diseases, lead, hazardous chemicals, radioactive material, excessive noise, extremes of temperature, or shock and vibration.

If there *is* a risk and your working conditions or hours can't be adjusted to protect you from it, your employer must find you suitable alternative work on the same terms and conditions. If that can't be done either, you should be suspended from work on paid leave, for as long as is necessary. If you're still concerned that your needs aren't being met, do speak up: chat directly to your boss, a human resources manager, or an employee rep, if you have one. If that doesn't get you anywhere, contact an organisation such as Citizens Advice, ACAS, or the Health and Safety Executive (HSE) for advice.

If you need help

In a nutshell, your rights to protection against risks, and for any necessary time off for antenatal care, must be upheld, and you cannot be discriminated against at work simply because you're having a baby. If for some reason you're unhappy with the way you've been treated by your employer, you should seek further advice from a relevant organisation or law company. We've listed some at the back of the book.

Coping with stress

If you do a job where anxiety levels are high, you may quite reasonably worry about the effect it could have on your baby. Fortunately, being fairly resilient little souls, unborn babies will generally weather most of the emotional storms life throws at you.

Severe or prolonged bouts of stress could raise your blood pressure, though, and that can cause complications in pregnancy. So if work-related worries are really causing you grief – especially if they're leading to physical problems, such as insomnia or headaches – then you might have to gently remind your employer about their legal responsibility to protect your health and safety while at work. They have a duty to remove any factors that are causing you stress, where possible, or adjust your conditions or hours accordingly.

If you don't feel you're getting the sympathy you need, chat to your midwife or doctor about it: they might want to sign you off for a while so you can get some rest. (Your boss might not like this – but they will have to lump it.)

Tired all the time?

Plain old exhaustion is one of the hardest things to deal with while working throughout pregnancy. Unfortunately, in most jobs at least, you need to remain in an upright position for the duration of your working day or shift, when in fact what you'd really like to do is lie down and nap. During the first trimester, surging hormones can cause an overpowering urge to sleep – and during the third, you might just lose the will to move altogether. Both problems are exacerbated if you're having trouble sleeping, which lots of pregnant women do. And, naturally, if you do a physical job, or are on your feet for a large part of the day, you'll probably have it even worse.

If you're struggling to get through the day, take a short lunchtime 'power nap' if need be (a snooze of about 15–20 minutes is ideal – any more than that and you may feel worse than when you started). In theory, employers have a duty to provide a place for you to rest, if possible, although in reality it may not be practicable. At the very least, a chair and a desk or other sur-face for you to lay your head down may be better than nothing.

You're likely to find you're fit for nothing but collapsing in a heap on the sofa when you get home after work. As *Modern Mum* Naomi recalls: 'I was so shocked by how utterly fatigued I felt during the first trimester particu-larly. I just collapsed at the end of the working day.'

Don't make any ambitious plans for weekday evenings if you can help it. Use the time to rest in front of a film, have a soak in the bath, get in some gentle stretches (or maybe even the odd massage from your other half), and get an early night whenever possible.

Be comfortable

Back and pelvic pain are common in pregnancy and can be made worse by sitting or standing for prolonged periods. You also increase your risk of deep vein thrombosis (see page 37) if you sit still for too long, and of dizziness or fainting when you stand. So it's vital to make sure you're as comfortable as you can be while working and that you take regular breaks either to move around or to sit down, as often as necessary. If you're on your feet, wear the most comfortable shoes you can bear. And if you're on your butt, be sure to take a short break from your workstation for a few moments, preferably at least once or twice an hour.

Make sure your desk and chair are positioned to give you maximum com-fort, too – you should ask for a new set-up if your existing one doesn't give you enough space or causes you discomfort that could otherwise be avoided (see the box below for more tips).

'We had those tall desks with high swivel chairs and it was super tricky to balance my beach ball middle on the top and not slide onto the floor. I got a lower desk eventually. Thank goodness. My work also involved a bit of air travel, which I was a bit over by the end.'

Kat

Are you sitting comfortably?

- Make sure your chair is high enough. Your feet should be flat on the floor with your hips slightly higher than your knees. Raise your feet if necessary with a box or stool.

- Your computer screen should be positioned directly in front of you.

- Give your spine support with a small cushion placed between the chair and the small of your back.

- Armrests can save the day if you're struggling to hoist yourself out of your chair – if you don't have them, ask your boss to provide them.

- Take regular breaks. Get up and move around for a couple of minutes, at least a couple of times an hour.

- Don't cross your legs – it will twist your spine and can affect the circulation. (In fact, get used to sitting like a bloke in the later stages – it's almost impossible to bring your knees together with a very big belly.

- Sit up straight, but with relaxed shoulders.

- Try to keep your pelvis tilted slightly upwards while you sit.

- You could also aim to fit in some daily ab-strengthening squeezes or pelvic floor exercises (see page 120) while you work.

Feeling sick

Whoever coined the term 'morning sickness' obviously hadn't suffered from it, since, usually, it goes on all day. Unfortunately, there's very little you can do to ease pregnancy nausea but in most cases it's mild (if relentless). There's more info and a few other ideas for coping with morning sickness on page 43.

'I had horrendous morning sickness, albeit never in the morning. A nausea worse than any hangover known to womankind would hit its peak between 5pm and 7pm (which made the commute home horrendous). I couldn't do much other than breathe deeply and hope it would pass, and it did – about six weeks later!'

Debbie

Some managers may be reluctant to make allowances for severe morning sickness (or for other pregnancy-related conditions, for that matter). But the law says they cannot discriminate against you in these circumstances – time off for pregnancy-related problems should be considered no different from any general sick leave (except if it happens in the last four weeks before you're due to start your leave, in which case your employer's entitled to clock you off for maternity leave as of then).

'I had to tell my line directors at work, as there was a two-week period in the first trimester when I did not go to the office because I was so sick.'

Beatriz

If you *do* need to take time off sick because you're ill in pregnancy and you get any grief about it, get a note from your midwife or GP, and stand firm. Remember, you cannot be threatened with discipline or sacking just for taking time off if you're ill through pregnancy. If you are, you could have a good case for an employment tribunal.

If you're suffering badly from nausea, you may find that it's the thing most likely to give you away while you're keeping your pregnancy a secret. Morning sickness in my first pregnancy put paid to my usual breakfast of a bacon butty and large black coffee – instead, my working day started with plain white toast and a Ribena. When, at 13 weeks, I made the official 'announcement' that I was pregnant, my colleagues rolled around laughing for a while before admitting they'd known for only slightly less time than I had.

'Preg head'

There's no conclusive scientific evidence for the existence of 'baby brain', but plenty of the anecdotal variety – ask any woman who's ever been pregnant and she'll no doubt have an example of how her mind went to mush. Theories vary and, in fact, the most recent research on the subject, by a team of experts from Australia, found that cognitive abilities are actually likely to *improve* during pregnancy.

Research aside, though, there's little doubt that, with so much on your mind, exhaustion rampaging through your body, and so many other physical symptoms distracting you, being pregnant can cause many a 'mind block'.

There's not a great deal to be done to combat 'preg head'. Keep a detailed to-do list in front of you at all times – and give yourself a break (literally and figuratively) whenever possible. If you're really struggling, you may need to enlist the sympathy of colleagues by explaining that your brain, as well as your body, has got a lot on right now.

‘I think probably my biggest work challenge was trying to prove I didn't have "baby brain" and could still do my job as well as before, balanced against wanting people to acknowledge that I was pregnant and more tired than usual.’

Julia

COPING WITH THE COMMUTE

When you're pregnant, getting to work and back can suddenly seem like the journey from (and to) hell. I cycled nearly every day until my third trimester weeks, when I had to start getting the train. Suddenly I was literally pressing my bump up against people on a crowded commuter train, and despite clearly being heavily pregnant and wearing my 'Baby on board!' badge, I still found that most commuters had selective blindness – they will not offer you a seat unless you ask them or stand in front of them sighing heavily and drumming your fingers on your bump. This can lead to bouts of late-pregnancy hormone-fuelled anger. So I'm told …

Do remember that, as part of your rights, your manager needs to ensure that you're not getting overtired or overstressed, so if the journey's really getting you down, you could reasonably request a change in start and finish times so you avoid the rush hour. If it's feasible, you could even ask for the chance to work from home a few days a week.

Public transport

Getting a seat on public transport is one of the great trials of pregnancy. Ironically, you won't get offered one when you might feel you need it most, in the first trimester, and for most of the second your fellow commuters will probably be so worried that you're simply overweight, rather than pregnant, they won't want to ask. Sadly, even being very obviously pregnant is no guarantee that someone will do the decent thing. If no-one's budging, just ask outright. London Underground can provide a 'Baby on board!' badge to bluntly alert other passengers to a pregnant woman's presence; they are available from London Underground's customer services department, or you can purchase one from eBay for the grand sum of 99p.

Top tips for commuting

- Leave home a little earlier (or later, if that works better) if it means you can avoid the worst of the rush hour. Even 15–30 minutes could make all the difference.

- Once you're showing, unbutton your coat and stick your belly out, so there's no doubt that you're in the family way.

- Be bold. Ask outright for a seat if you feel you need one.

- Wear a 'Baby on board!' badge.

- Don't leave home without a snack and a bottle of water in your bag. You may need sustenance if you feel faint or poorly.

Driving

If you drive to work, make sure you're as comfortable as you can be in the driving seat. If your back hurts, you might get a bit of relief from a small cushion supporting your lower back. Break the journey up to stretch your legs if it's a long one. And once you've got a reasonable-sized bump, consider investing in a 'bump belt'. This is a cushioned strap that can be easily attached, and detached, from your seat belt, keeping it in a position underneath your bump and allowing a safer and more comfortable ride for you and your baby.

IF YOUR BOSS IS BEING A BUGGER

Some companies are enlightened and experienced in matters of maternity – others aren't. And even if your manager is technically playing the game, you may still be suffering from more resentful attitudes or a lack of support, which can be upsetting. 'My boss was always hard work but he became worse when I was pregnant – everything was my fault,' reveals *Modern Mum* Marie. 'He knew how to push those buttons and I nearly walked on more than one occasion. I took the matter up with the other partners and the issue was resolved, thankfully.'

If there's no higher level of management you can go to, try to rise above any less-than-helpful mindsets by focusing on doing your job as best you can, thinking about your baby, and reminding yourself that it's a short-term period in your life with an end goal that overrides everything else. Like Marie, make a pledge to yourself that you won't let the bastards get you down. 'There were times when my work was affected by my terrible morning sickness,' she says, 'but I carried on regardless.'

Above all, remind yourself that the law is on your side: if you're not happy with the way you're being treated, swot up on your rights and don't be afraid to share that information with your boss, if you need to.

WANT TO GO BACK TO YOUR CAREER?

Although you may not be ready yet to make a decision about what the future holds for you, workwise, it's something to think about. And even if you do have fairly firm ideas at this stage – maybe you know for certain you don't want to go back at all, or maybe you feel very sure that full-time motherhood is definitely not your bag – remember that many women change their minds once they've dropped their sprog and have spent a bit of time with the little ankle-biter. Have a general game plan in mind, by all means – but remain open-minded, too.

If you know or think that you're going back to work at some point after your baby's birth, one thing you will need to sort out is some reliable childcare. It's never too early to be looking into this, since popular nurseries and childminders in busy areas often have waiting lists, and you'll need to know about costs if you've got budgeting to do. We've included some useful contact details for organisations concerned with childcare at the back of the book.

'Keeping in touch' days

If you're so minded, and if your employer is keen for you to do so, you can spend up to 10 days in your workplace, for which you can be paid, during maternity leave. Known as 'keeping in touch' days, these offer a chance for you to keep up with what's going on at work and maintain links with your colleagues. They don't have to be spent doing your usual job but could involve training or some other special event. Some women find them a useful way of dipping their toes back into their jobs after a long spell away. 'Keeping in touch' days are by no means compulsory, though, from either your point of view or your boss's.

Equally, your employer is entitled to make 'reasonable contact' with you while you're away, if they need to refer to you about a work matter that just can't wait. But they cannot demand that you go into work for any reason – that's down to you.

'I really regret not going to my 'keeping in touch' days – when I finally returned after over a year I felt like a fish out of water.'

Rowan

Returning to work after maternity leave

You must give your employer 28 days' notice if you plan to return to work before the end of Ordinary Maternity Leave (in other words, during the first 26 weeks of your year's entitlement), or eight weeks' notice if you plan to go back during Additional Maternity Leave (that is, during the second 26 weeks). If you go back before the Ordinary Maternity Leave period is up, you're entitled to go back to the same job you had before leaving to have your baby. If you go back during your Additional Maternity Leave, you should either get your old job back or be offered something else where the terms and conditions are just as good.

'I would say the minute you start your maternity leave you should update your CV and review your skills. Once you start to think about it after having your baby, your brain has turned to mush. It's so much better to do it while it's fresh in your mind.'

Melissa

If you decide not to go back to work at all, you have to give your employer whatever notice period your contract demands – it would make sense to do this so that your official leaving date coincides with the end of your maternity leave, to save having to go back for a short period to work out your notice. You won't have to pay back any statutory maternity pay, but, if your company has paid you more than the statutory level under enhanced maternity benefits, they could ask you to pay all of it, or some of it, back.

'I'm very torn taking my maternity pay,' admits *Modern Mum* Nicola. 'I'm really not sure if I want to go back to work after I finish maternity leave, but I know I'll have to save rather than spend the money as I might have to pay it back!' You may also decide you want to request a return to work with shorter hours or a more flexible set-up.

'On the one hand at work, the news was greeted with great happiness and support. I was offered flexibility, my colleagues were very caring, it was very pleasant. On the other hand, yes, there were comments and attitudes that were definitely sexist. The main problem is that these comments were kind of innocent, naive. Attitudes are so ingrained that no-one believes they are being patronising when, for instance, they decide they know how you will feel once the baby is born. Yes, I will feel different; I have no idea whether I will want to return to work full time, or part time, or not return at all. I think I know, but I DON'T. But you wouldn't know either. So do not tell me how I will feel. Do not tell me how I will think!'

Beatriz

Requesting flexible working

Lots of women find that returning to work, but part time or on a more flexible basis than before (either with fewer days, shorter hours or work-from-home opportunities, perhaps), gives them the work–life balance they're looking for. There's no law that says you *must* be given flexible work if you want it, but anyone who's been with an employer for 26 weeks and who has a child under 16 (dads, too) is entitled to request it – and their manager must give it 'serious consideration'. You've nothing to lose by asking.

'Work was very tiring towards the end. Commuting was pretty rubbish and the evening work was just exhausting. However, I was in a good streak professionally and they wanted me back – on my terms – so that was really satisfying.'

Natalie

WHEN YOU'RE THE BOSS

If you run your own company or work for yourself, it will be down to you to decide how long you go on working for and how much time you take off with your baby. You'll probably need to sit down, do some sums, and ask yourself some questions: for example, can you survive on Maternity Allowance, and, if so, for how long? You'll also be responsible for taking care of yourself, and ensuring your own health and safety. Of course, the upside of being your own boss during pregnancy is that if you do really need to spend the morning with your head in a bucket, or switch off your computer and take a nap after lunch, you (usually) can.

6 Hit and missionary

Your pregnant love life

GAGGING FOR IT OR JUST GAGGING?

It's what got you into this state in the first place. Yet, ironically, sex can become a little scarce in the nine months that follow conception. A very normal experience for women in pregnancy is to have a distinct dearth of bedroom action in the first trimester, as sickness and exhaustion take their toll; a fairly fruity second trimester, as you begin to feel human again and (in some cases) the so-called pregnancy 'horn' takes hold; and a return to the drought during the third, since making love when you're the size of an elephant – and about as flexible – tends to lose its appeal. It doesn't always work that way, of course. Some women find that their sex drive remains unimpaired throughout pregnancy. Others are virtually celibate for the duration.

'One of the best things about my pregnancy was the sex! My partner and I have always had great sex but the orgasms were mind-blowing for most of the first two trimesters. My partner felt like a rock star.'

Jenn

'I definitely felt more connected to my husband – it felt like a very special thing we were experiencing together. I also felt more comfortable and confident in my body – much happier to be naked. However, I did feel nervous about sex, and between the sickness in the mornings and tiredness at night it was tough to find time for it.'

Julie

143

Why you might not want to have sex when you're pregnant

- You feel too sick.

- You feel too tired.

- You feel fat, and you're self-conscious about it.

- Your piles/back/pelvis/tits/bladder hurt too much (delete as appropriate, or leave all).

- You're worried it could be harmful to your baby.

- You're worried in general. And stressed. And tearful. In short, you're not in the mood.

- You *have actually* got a headache.

- You can't bear the way your other half smells anymore.

'My long-suffering husband has had to deal with virtually no sex during both my pregnancies – the idea of having sex is not altogether unwelcome, but at the end of a long day sleep is my number one priority. Anyway, sex is what got me into this mess in the first place.'

Becca

Pregnancy sex myth busted!

The big 'O' won't bring on premature labour! You may experience mild contractions when you orgasm, which can feel a little weird, but they won't be strong enough to trigger labour, unless your body's all ready to go in any case.

IS HE HORNY? DO YOU CARE?!

Of course, pregnancy can alter the way men feel about sex, too. It's not unusual for a bloke to be scared, repelled or just a bit freaked out by the thought because you've got his baby inside you. Some blokes even have a genuine fear of poking the baby's head with their willy. All very well if you're not much in the mood yourself. Rather unfortunate if you happen to be gagging for it.

Pregnancy sex myth busted!

Your partner's penis – however big it may be – will never ever make contact with your baby! The angle of the vagina means that there's no way his willy will bump the baby, unless he has a 90-degree kink in his love tackle; it's anatomically impossible.

Why he may not want to have sex when you're pregnant

- He's also worried it could be harmful to the baby.
- His child is inside you: it's just too weird!
- You're a mother now, or about to be. You've ceased to be a sexual being to him.

'We carried on as normal for the first few months, which was great, but once my bump became quite noticeable my husband felt quite uncomfortable, so we just stopped having sex.'

Jo

Pregnancy sex myth busted!

The baby won't get squashed! He's very well cushioned in his amniotic sac, and will be completely untroubled by your bedroom antics.

MAKE SEX WORK

Sex in pregnancy can be a good thing, so, if you *can* maintain a sex life for some of the nine months, there are lots of benefits to be had. For instance:

- There's no need to fumble for a condom or fret that you forgot your pill.
- Increased blood flow to the pelvic region can mean faster, bigger and better orgasms.
- Your boobs may be a growing attraction.
- It will make you feel emotionally close to each other.
- You don't have much choice but to experiment with sexual positions.
- It's good exercise for your pelvic muscles in preparation for birth.
- It's sex purely for the heck of it (perhaps relevant if you had fertility issues, and were more concerned with making a baby than making love).
- It will make you feel relaxed and sleepy – the perfect antidote to stress and insomnia.
- It might just help move things along if you're due or overdue.
- Once the baby's born, you probably won't make love for ages. In other words, *get some now, while you still can ...!*

Pregnancy sex myth busted!

Having sex won't cause you to have a miscarriage! Although, if you've had one before or you've had some bleeding, your doctor or midwife might advise you to abstain, just to be on the safe side.

The pregnancy horn

Higher levels of hormones and an increased blood flow in the pelvic area mean it all becomes a bit swollen and super-sensitive down there and thus

– in theory – faster arousal and better, longer orgasms. (Presumably this is Mother Nature's little apology for the host of horrors she's inflicted elsewhere on your body.) However, plenty of women don't experience any more stirrings down below than is normal – I know I didn't, sadly.

There's also a flipside to this particular pregnancy 'perk': the area can become *too* sensitive, making arousal and orgasm uncomfortable. Boobs, too, can be affected by a hormonal blood rush, and may feel unbearably sore.

‘Sexually, I went a bit rampant. I was feeling extraordinarily mother-earthy and invigorated and fancied the pants off him even more.’

Nicki

Oral sex

Making love doesn't have to mean penetration – even if you don't fancy full-on sex, you don't have to give up on intimacy. You could still have quite a lot of fun with some good, old-fashioned mutual masturbation, and oral sex doesn't take much effort – especially if it's him on you. One thing might affect this, though: hormonal influences can make your vaginal secretions heavier than usual, and they could smell and taste a bit different. Of course, there's no particular reason why you can't return the favour – except perhaps if you feel sick, have a funny taste in your mouth, can't abide the smell of just about anything, or cannot actually bend over because your back hurts or your belly's getting in the way …

Pregnancy sex myth busted!

Cunnilingus will not kill you! Boy-on-girl oral sex is perfectly safe. However, just in case he was considering it, don't let your partner blow hard inside you. There's a small risk, in theory, that it could cause an air bubble to enter your circulatory system and lead to a potentially fatal embolism.

Other ways of being intimate

Of course, you don't even have to get sexy to get intimate. A massage or a simple naked cuddle can feel pretty good and will help remind you that you're a couple, and not just two people sharing a bed who are about to have a baby together.

Finding a comfortable position

Straightforward missionary ceases to be comfortable once you've got a significant belly on you – not only will it get in the way, but lying flat on your back can put pressure on the main vein, and that can cause dizziness. A pillow under your bottom should raise your lower back enough to prevent this, and if you position yourself right on the edge of the bed and get your man to stand (or kneel), you'll be sorted.

Woman-on-top isn't a bad alternative either, although it does mean you've got to do the work, which isn't ideal if you're tired, and he'll have a serious eyeful of your belly, which you may feel self-conscious about. For variation, you could try this sitting on a chair (make sure it's a strong one).

Best of all is probably anything with a behind-entry theme: 'doggy style' with you on your hands and knees can work well. If that doesn't appeal there's the gentler version, 'spoons', where you lie down together on your sides, facing the same way, with him behind you.

You'll have to use your imaginations a bit when it comes to sex in late pregnancy – chances are you'll try out more positions during pregnancy than you did in your first three months together. A sense of humour, and a selection of pillows, may help.

Pregnancy sex myth busted!

The baby won't be exposed to an infection! The thick mucus plug that seals off the cervix means bacteria can't get through, and your baby is perfectly safe.

Keep talking

It's totally normal for one or both halves of a couple to go off sex for some reason during pregnancy, and that's fine. Any half-decent partner – however sex-starved – should be able to see it as a temporary phase in the context of your whole lives together. The fact that there might not be much sex around for a while after you've had the baby is neither here nor there. Sex lives do tend to get put on hold when you first become parents, but, fortunately, they almost always come back again.

If things are lacking in the bedroom department, it's a really good idea to talk about why, if you can, and to make sure that there are plenty of kisses, cuddles and touching to make up for it. It's all too easy to feel rejected when your partner doesn't want sex with you, even if they do have a damn good excuse for not being much in the mood, so it's important to make sure the 'unwilling' party lets the other one know they still care.

❛I loved my new curves, bigger boobs, a reason to have a belly. All the new blood in my body made everything more fun! We had lots of sex throughout my pregnancy, right up to the end.❜

Hannah

BRINGING ON LABOUR

It's a well-worn piece of advice that making love when your baby is due is a good way to kick-start proceedings. There is some scientific basis for this, which is probably why most expectant couples give it at least one shot in the closing weeks (when, in fact, for many women sex is the least important thing on their minds).

The hormone oxytocin, which is also called the 'love hormone', is released during orgasm and makes the womb contract and helps 'limber up' the cervix ready for its big role in birth. Added to that, semen contains prostaglandin, a hormone-like substance which is said to soften the cervix. Prolonged bouts of nipple fondling can also encourage a release of oxytocin – however, you do have to fondle them for quite long periods if this is really going to work (see page 206). And why ever not?

You shouldn't have sex if your waters are leaking, or if you've had a 'show' (see page 203), which means the mucus plug sealing your cervix has come away, or partly come away, as it could leave your baby vulnerable to infection.

Pregnancy sex myth busted!

The baby has no idea you are shagging! He might have an idea something exciting's afoot because your heartbeat's all over the place – and he'll hear you, if you've a tendency to be 'vocal' about these things. And yes, he might even decide to get in on the act by kicking and moving around a bit. But he doesn't know you're at it. Really.

WHEN NOT TO HAVE SEX

Your doctor or midwife might suggest you give sex a miss during one or more parts of your pregnancy if they reckon it could be risky: for instance, if you've a history of miscarriage, have suffered bleeding, your waters have burst early, or if you have or could have placenta praevia (see page 15). Hold off sex until you've spoken to your midwife if you do experience any amount of bleeding – even though it may be due to something harmless such as cervical ectropion (see page 67), it should always be investigated.

Some sexually transmitted diseases, such as genital herpes, syphilis, gonorrhoea, HIV and chlamydia, could infect your baby either in the womb or during delivery, and prove seriously harmful to him. If you suspect you're carrying one of these – or that your partner is – let your midwife or doctor know straight away so they can arrange for testing and treatment.

LOOKING AFTER YOUR RELATIONSHIP

It's not just the physical side of your love life that's affected by pregnancy. It can be a challenging time emotionally, too. You may have numerous symptoms to cope with – none of which he can do anything about, or have any inkling of the extent of their awfulness – as well as unpredictable mood swings that you must both contend with.

The upshot of that may well be large doses of resentment. 'My relationship did go through some really rough patches,' says Becca. 'My husband decided that he needed to go out and get hammered every weekend as this might be his "last" opportunity. Even though I reminded him that half the guys he was going out with already had children …'

While you seethe, he's probably feeling frustrated, since his attempts to help are, more than likely, ungratefully received. On top of all that, both of you are likely to be anxious about whether your baby will be okay, the birth, and the huge responsibility that lies ahead as parents. And, with a child to provide for and a partner who may not be earning for a while, he could well be feeling the pressure of being the main breadwinner. Add in the fact that your sex life may not be going with a swing, and you can see why pregnancy can put a strain on even the strongest of relationships. The best thing you can do to keep your love for each other ticking over healthily during pregnancy is to talk to each other.

Silence can breed resentment, so try to let him know (preferably in a calm and measured way, rather than screaming) how you're feeling. Although he will never truly know what hell you are going through in order to bring his child into the world, you can make sure he's got some idea by thrusting an informative guide such as this one in his hand.

'I did sometimes think that my husband forgot that I was pregnant and just thought I was getting tired for no reason. I really wanted him to give up drinking or give up something as I was having to do. I guess that did make me feel a bit resentful -- like I'm the one doing all the hard work and his life can continue as normal.'

Julia

Talking's a two-way street, of course, so make sure you extend an ear to his woes too. If you're arguing more than usual, be sure to kiss and make up before things get out of hand. And pencil in as many slots as possible to spend with each other. Discuss your plans for the birth and for parenthood, and talk about the changing phases of your pregnancy by all means. But sometimes it's a good idea to put the whole pregnancy/baby thing out of the equation for a while and talk about something completely different.

Try, too, to give each other a bit of space where necessary. Aim to spend time with people other than your other half – and encourage him to do his own thing too. Above all, try to keep in mind that pregnancy is a temporary phase in any couple's shared lifetime. Happily, most people find that, ultimately, pregnancy and parenthood bring them closer together, not further apart.

'My husband was pretty much as great as a man could be (even during my moody hormonal moments) but I still had times when I felt he didn't really get it.'

Natalie

Any problems you're up against now will usually fade into insignificance once your baby's born and it becomes clear that what you've been through was a means to a wonderful end. (Of course, having a new baby can also put all sorts of pressures on a couple's love life – but that's another subject.)

If your relationship really seems in trouble, it would be a good idea to thrash things out before the baby's arrival. You might want to consider some couples counselling, through an organisation such as Relate. There are some useful addresses at the back of the book.

7 Delivery schedule

Making plans for your baby's arrival

Unless you're in total denial, you'll want to give plenty of advance thought to the momentous event that comes right at the end of pregnancy. Birth can be a pretty nerve-racking prospect, especially when it's your first baby and you don't have much else apart from other people's birth stories and scary scenes from *One Born Every Minute* to go by. But one thing's certain: this baby's coming out of you, and you need to be prepared for it.

While you can never really know what birth's like until you've actually been through it, you can help yourself be ready for it by doing your 'homework' (reading this book will be a good start).

The important thing to bear in mind is that where birth's concerned – particularly your first – nothing's guaranteed. So when it comes to planning yours, you should keep an open mind until the time comes. It's kind of like planning a picnic in the British summer – make the plans expecting sunshine, but be prepared that there's always a chance it'll rain.

Obviously, it's a good idea to be prepared by knowing as much as possible about having a baby. In particular (while you certainly shouldn't worry yourself unduly about them), there are all sorts of things that can occur during labour and birth that require special treatment, and it's a good idea to know in advance what they are so that, should anything happen during yours, you'll be well informed and confident about things. Chapter 9 of this book tells you all you need to know about the basics of birth – so make sure you look at it well in advance of your due date, rather than saving it as reading material for labour.

WHERE YOU'RE GOING TO HAVE YOUR BABY

There are three basic options when it comes to where you're going to give birth:

- consultant-led hospital unit
- midwife-led (or GP-led) unit
- home birth.

As this is a pretty important decision and could have quite a big impact on how your birth turns out, you'd be wise to give it some thought. What follows is a broad outline, but there's lots more detail at www.which.co.uk/birth-choice, an impartial website offering loads of information on the choices you need to make, and what's available in your area.

Once you've made a decision about where to give birth, you don't have to stick to it. You're entitled to change your mind at any point.

CONSULTANT-LED HOSPITAL UNIT

The majority of women choose a consultant-led hospital maternity unit. And although there's no doubt that some can seem a bit grim – often with peeling paint and a selection of scary-looking items of equipment – they do offer the reassurance of access to the whole gamut of pain-relief options, and any medical aids that may be required. There'll always be an obstetrician on call if needed during the pregnancy or birth, and you'll be in the best place should an emergency arise. All of which is probably why, for the vast majority of mums, a hospital maternity unit seems the most appealing place to have your baby the first time round.

Once you're booked in, you may be offered a chance to take a look round the maternity unit. While this can be reassuring and informative, it may also leave you feeling a bit wobbly – just like *Modern Mum* Isla. 'I visited the hospital at 25 weeks,' she says. 'There were bars on the side of the bed and it felt like I was walking onto the set of *One Flew Over the Cuckoo's Nest*. Luckily the same hospital had a gorgeous birthing unit downstairs, with a pool, and I decided to go there instead.' Some hospitals no longer offer tours, however, due to health and safety reasons, and many offer online tours instead!

If you do visit your chosen maternity ward, use it as a chance to ask questions and familiarise yourself with basic stuff, such as where the loos and nearest catering facilities are – let's face it, when the time comes to check in for real, you'll have other stuff on your mind. You can also find out what potentially useful equipment there is available: for instance, a birthing pool, aids such as birthing balls, comfy cushions or bean bags, a CD player or iPod dock. Delivery rooms these days tend to be more comfortable and better equipped for birth than they used to be. But if not, you might be able to bring what you need with you.

MIDWIFE-LED UNIT

In some areas, and providing you're not at high risk of some complication arising during birth, you may also be offered the option of having your baby in the more 'homely' setting of a midwife-led maternity unit, sometimes called a GP-led unit, or a birthing centre. These usually operate independently, but some are attached to hospitals. There are growing numbers of these sorts of units, but not every area has one yet.

Because they're staffed by midwives, you won't see any scary-looking forceps-wielding consultants in green coats in a birthing centre. The focus is more likely to be on a relaxed and natural experience, and it certainly seems to pan out that way in most cases – statistics show that women who have their babies in this kind of unit are less likely to need assistance in the form of vacuum extraction (ventouse) or forceps (see page 222), or to go on to have a caesarean section (see pages 174 and 224).

Birthing centres are equipped with the things that make natural birth more of a possibility – water pools, for example – and are likely to be more comfortable all round, a 'home away from home' vibe. There may also be room for your other half to stay in there with you. But there won't be an obstetrician or anaesthetist immediately to hand, which means you won't get an epidural here (something you might regret when you realise just how effing painful your natural birth has turned out to be), and there are no facilities for surgery or for special baby care. And, of course, in the event of certain emergencies, you'd still face the inconvenience of being transferred by ambulance to the nearest appropriate hospital – although, in some cases, that will be right next door or up a couple of floors in a lift, which is reassuring.

HOME BIRTH

If you're very hospital-averse, or simply determined to do the whole darn thing as nature intended, you might want to consider giving birth in the comfort and privacy of your own home (although you might want to let your neighbours know there could be some screaming going on and not to call the police ...). When things go right, your own home is the perfect place to have your baby. I know plenty of *Modern Mums* who've popped one out in their lounge only to be tucked up half an hour later under their own duvet, eating pizza and snuggling with their newborn. Being at home and in a familiar environment is said to reduce stress, and less stress means less of the 'fight or flight' hormone adrenaline, which equals a smoother, swifter labour. You will also be under the care of just one or two community midwives, who'll stick with you throughout the whole experience, rather than subject to the changing shift patterns of the average maternity unit.

But there's absolutely no doubt about the drawbacks of this option. If anything happens that's beyond the capabilities of the midwife who's with you, you'll be bundled into an ambulance faster than you can say 'epidural', and whisked off to your nearest hospital, blue lights ablaze. Not only that, but you won't have anything more than gas and air (see page 163) at your disposal for pain relief (although some midwives will administer pethidine, see page 165). As you'll see later in more detail, giving birth is really bloody painful indeed – and when it's your first, it can be prolonged, which means you can start off coping okay with the contractions but, 24 hours later, find that biting your lip and breathing is no longer enough for you.

An average of 2.5% of babies in the UK are born at home, which is a small number, but that figure breaks down interestingly: approximately 1 in 30 in Wales, 1 in 40 in England, 1 in 165 in Scotland, and 1 in 250 in Northern Ireland.

If a woman wants to have her baby at home and there are no obvious major risks involved, then she should certainly be able to. In theory, the choice is open to all women, although, in reality, there are still some areas where you might be discouraged, or even told outright it won't be possible, with staff shortages or cutbacks usually given the blame.

And wherever you live, you're likely to be discouraged from having a home birth if there's any complicating factor that means you'd be safer giving birth in a hospital: for instance, if you have a medical condition such as pre-eclampsia, if you're expecting twins, or if your baby's in the breech position as you come close to your due date. Some health professionals are even pretty categorical in their belief that home birth isn't a sensible option for *any* woman giving birth for the first time (but the risk is considerably diminished with a second birth).

Anecdotally, of my *Modern Mums* interviewed for this book, about one in five had a home birth (a couple of them accidentally!). So it's definitely becoming more of an accepted option.

Do have a good read up on the subject if home birth is something you'd like to look into (I've included some sympathetic resources at the back of the book). And if you want to go for it, go for it.

Some home-birthers opt to hire an independent midwife so they can get comprehensive support. This is a pretty expensive option (fees range from

£2,000 to £4,500), but women who have done so usually report high levels of satisfaction. There's more information on the website of the Independent Midwives Association.

MAKING A BIRTH PLAN

Once you know where you're having your baby, it's a good idea to make some more specific plans for the sort of birth you want – or rather, that you hope for. Things to think about include pain relief, birthing positions, and stuff that you might prefer to avoid, *if possible*. What isn't a good idea is having a rigid idea of how you want things to pan out because, ultimately, you don't know what fate has in store for you on the day and how you'll cope with it. So plan by all means, but don't laminate your birth plan and imagine those plans to be set in stone. Promise yourself you'll see what happens when the time comes.

Many people would argue that 'making a birth plan' is as futile a use of a pregnant woman's time as shopping for stilettos: you simply cannot 'plan' what's going to happen during your labour. But still, there's no harm in considering your utopia. If you do have any feelings one way or another about how – in an ideal world – you'd like your baby's birth to go, it's worth getting it down on paper. At the very least, it will help you confront the issues that are likely to arise.

During labour, assuming there's time, your midwife should be happy to take a look at yours and to do what she can to abide by your wishes as far as is possible. On the other hand, there's always the possibility that it never makes it out of the bag …

'I don't think anyone or anything can fully prepare you for labour, partly because it is so different for everyone. So I'm not sure it would've helped that much if I'd really known the extent of how hard it would be. Nothing else in life gives you anything close to that kind of reward though.'

Anna

Above all, remember this: if you do make a birth plan, there's no point in making any inflexible pledges or demands, because you just don't know what's going to happen and how you'll cope. Avoid statements like 'I absolutely refuse to have this baby taken out of me surgically', for example, or 'Strap me to the bed and inject the epidural on my arrival'. Instead, stick to phrases like 'I hope to avoid a delivery by ventouse or forceps and would like to be given time to consider measures such as these if thought necessary.' And do cover all eventualities, if you can. When I wrote mine the first time, I was canny enough to predict that I'd be begging for an epidural and made sure I mentioned it in the plan, just in case I was rendered incoherent with pain and unable to ask for one. Quite rightly, as it turned out.

If you're not sure what to put in your birth plan, there are some ideas below. You'll also find some good advice on the NHS Choices and BabyCentre websites. Some maternity units even provide a printed form to help you get your plan on paper. Make sure it's typed or written neatly, so that the midwife can actually make sense of it. And do share it with your antenatal care team. They'll be able to let you know if there's anything about your personal circumstances that might be relevant.

What you might want to include if you make a birth plan

- The sort of pain relief you think you want – and any that you'd quite like to avoid.

- Who your birth partner's going to be.

- What sort of positions you're keen to try out – for instance, if you think you'd prefer to be standing or kneeling to have your baby and whether you'd like to remain active if possible.

- Whether you'd like to give the birthing pool a whirl, if they have one.

- Any desire you may have to avoid certain procedures – induction, or an episiotomy, for example – if at all possible.

- Whether or not you're happy to have an injection to speed up the delivery of the placenta.

- If your partner is keen to cut the umbilical cord, and whether you want it to stop pulsing before it's cut.

- How you plan to feed your baby, if you want to breastfeed, and if you want skin-to-skin contact with your baby immediately, before they clean her up.

Of course, for many women, a birth plan may amount to nothing more than the following phrase: 'I am happy for you to do whatever it takes to help me give birth to my baby safely.' And that's an eminently sensible view.

HOPING FOR A 'NATURAL BIRTH'?

Definitions of natural birth vary, but it basically means going through labour and delivery without intervention or pain relief (other than things like massage, water or breathing techniques – and gas and air's usually considered allowable too, under 'natural birth' rules).

Certainly, there are advantages to a natural birth: research suggests you're more likely to have less postnatal pain and a faster recovery. Some people say that it's a more rewarding way to have a baby, which means you're more likely to look back on your birth with a sense of achievement. And some say it makes for easier bonding with your child, and more chance of successful breastfeeding.

Natural birth is an emotive issue. Many people believe that, if women were left to their own devices with the help of a supportive midwife, far more births could be natural than currently are, and far less intervention could be carried out. These people may well be right. But the truth is you're often too bewildered, scared or exhausted to do anything other than put your faith in the professionals. And it may well be that all you really care about, at that point, is for your baby to be born in one piece.

By all means plan for a natural birth. But try not to see it as the only outcome you'll be happy with. Don't think for a minute that you'll somehow have failed at your birth experience if it turns out not to be a 'natural' one. The truth is that sometimes it's *just not possible* to have a natural birth.

What you can do to improve your chances

- Read as much as you can. Look for Ina May Gaskin's *Ina May's Guide to Childbirth* (Vermilion, 2008) – she's a midwife guru who has delivered thousands of babies without a hint of intervention. Or try a lovely book called *Baby Catcher* (Simon & Schuster, 2003) by a US midwife called Peggy Vincent. *Birth Skills* (Vermilion, 2008) by Juju Sundin is another great source of information. Read and absorb as much as you can about birth and birthing techniques. Knowledge is power, and nowadays birthing 'naturally' is ironically something that we seem to have lost the natural ability to do without a bit of preparation and determination.

- Research having a home birth, or going to a midwife-led birthing centre. Having your baby in hospital doesn't mean you automatically forgo your chances of a natural birth (although, statistically, it does definitely reduce your chances). Make it clear that's what you'd like in your birth plan – and make sure your birth partner's fully briefed so they can pipe up during labour.

- Sign up for NCT antenatal classes, where the focus is usually slanted in favour of natural or low-intervention birth, and you can learn breathing and relaxation techniques. You could also look into alternative private antenatal courses such as active birth classes or antenatal yoga.

- Consider a water birth. Research has shown that women who spend part of their labour in a birthing pool are less likely to go on to have pain relief such as pethidine or an epidural, and there's also evidence that it can reduce the likelihood of tearing or needing an episiotomy. Some women use water in the first stage only, for pain relief, and get out to actually deliver their baby. But others choose to have their baby in the pool. There's more about water as a method of pain relief on page 168.

- Look into alternative methods of pain relief and relaxation such as hypnobirthing, acupuncture, aromatherapy, massage and breathing techniques (see page 167).

- Choose another woman as your birth partner. Research shows that having a female companion in the delivery room with you improves your likelihood of having a birth without intervention.

'I didn't really want Joe coming too close to me – I was happier with the midwives. Not sure if it was some kind of instinctive trust of other women when you're in that scenario or simply the fact that they knew what they were doing.'

Natalie

- If he's not there already, encourage your baby into the right position prior to birth (see page 200).

- Prepare for active birth positions such as standing up or kneeling, where gravity works with you to help your baby's descent down the birth canal. You'll be more confident about using them during the birth itself if you've tried them out beforehand.

'I ended up having a completely natural, no drugs water birth. Beforehand I was the first person to put their hand up and say, "Give me the drugs, I want the drugs!" But when it came to it, my labour went very smoothly and at no stage did I ever feel like things weren't progressing as they should do.'

Laura

PAIN RELIEF OPTIONS

Having a baby hurts. Quite how much it hurts, how long it will hurt for, and how you personally cope with the pain are all factors that it's impossible to generalise about. One thing that really changed the way I looked at labour pain was that it is a totally natural productive pain. It's not the pain from a bikini wax – it's *your* pain, unique to your body, your baby, your birth. In this respect, no amount of reading other people's opinions or experiences of pain can dictate how you will feel or react on the day. It's your pain, and it's there to bring your baby into the world.

Fortunately for modern women, medical science now offers us a number of pain relief options. Lots of women make it through birth without, either through choice or because circumstances dictate (if your baby comes in a hurry and there just isn't time, for example). But in the majority of births, pain relief of some kind is used.

Do your research and have a good, hard think about the type of pain relief you think will be right for you. And by all means write it down in your birth plan, if you want to. But whatever you decide, be totally and utterly prepared to change your mind (or to have it changed for you) when the time comes. You just cannot predict how intense, how prolonged and how bearable the pain is going to be.

Entonox – gas and air

What is it?

Gas and air, a mix of 50% oxygen and 50% nitrous oxide, is administered through a mouthpiece or mask from which you breathe it in. It's readily accessible and you're in control – chances are that when no-one's looking, your birth partner will demand a toke too.

When can I have some?

Any time during labour and birth, and whenever you feel the need. Since it also comes in portable canisters, it's one of the few forms of pain relief you can rely on if you're giving birth at home. You'll also be able to use it if you're giving birth in water, unlike most other forms of pain relief.

Is it any good?

It's one of the least powerful forms of pain relief for birth, but it can certainly take the edge off, so it's a good option in the earlier phases before the going gets tough. As it can take up to a minute for the effects to kick in, it's best to take it when you feel a contraction coming, rather than right in the middle of one.

Are there any drawbacks?

Gas and air creates a sort of 'high' that can render you woozy, like being really drunk – a sensation that might make you feel a bit out of control. It can also lead to a dry mouth and can sometimes make you feel nauseous. Otherwise, it has no adverse effects and is safe for you and your baby.

TENS machine

What is it?

A TENS (transcutaneous electrical nerve stimulation) machine is a little box which emits electrical pulses through four wires and four sticky pads, which you fix to your back. It works by intercepting pain signals to your brain, and by stimulating the release of endorphins, the body's natural pain-busting hormones. They have dials with which you can control the frequency and intensity of the pulses – start off low and increase them as the contractions get stronger.

When can I have some?

As early as you like – as it takes up to an hour for your body to respond, you should make sure you get it on in good time. You'll probably want to take it off towards the later stages of labour, as it's unlikely to help with very strong contractions and all the wires will just be a nuisance. You'll need some help from your birth partner or midwife to stick the pads on in the right place. You can't use a TENS machine in a birthing pool. Electric shocks and all that.

Is it any good?

Opinions vary – some women find them helpful, others say they're not particularly effective. Personally, I would say that they are great for managing the initial contractions but they won't even break the seal when the heavy mob moves in.

'I loved the TENS machine – it was such a good distraction in the early stages of labour and seemed to make the contractions bearable.'

Manna

What are the drawbacks?

I turned the voltage up too high by mistake on mine, causing a pulse so strong it made me squeal. You won't be able to get a back massage, either, as the pads will get in the way. TENS machines aren't routinely available in maternity units – although some NHS trusts lend them out – so if you want one you'll probably need to buy or hire it. They're available from a whole range of places, including specialist companies and from big shops such as Boots or Mothercare. Expect to pay between £20 and £30 to hire, and around £50–£70 to buy.

Painkilling drugs such as pethidine, meptid and diamorphine

What is it?

These painkilling drugs (also known as analgesics) are usually given via an injection in the thigh or bum, or occasionally direct into the bloodstream through a fine tube inserted into a vein in your arm. Midwives are able to administer them, so there'll be no need to call in a doctor if you want some. You may also be able to take control of your own dosage if the unit has a PCA (patient-controlled analgesia) device. Pethidine is the most widely used, while meptid and diamorphine are only available in some units. Check in advance what's available in yours.

When can I have some?

You can have any of these at any point, except when you're coming close to the pushing stage, as they're more likely to have a harmful effect on your baby if given too late in labour. You may be able to have pethidine at a home birth, but many midwives are reluctant to administer it because of the risks to the baby – it can be transferred to the baby's bloodstream and can make her drowsy.

Is it any good?

Reports from women vary – some say they were effective, others that they were little or no help in relieving the pain, although they usually make it easier to rest and relax between contractions.

What are the drawbacks?

They can make you feel very drowsy, dizzy or sick. If too much is given, or they're given too late, these sorts of drugs can hang around in your baby's system for several days after the birth, which could slow down her breathing and cause her to be very sleepy, perhaps affecting her feeding.

Epidural

What is it?

An anaesthetic injection into the space around the spine, which numbs the nerve supply that serves the uterus and cervix giving complete, and fast, relief from pain. Although quite a lot of women say they'd rather avoid one when planning a first birth, quite a lot end up having one: around a quarter. Some hospitals offer a mobile epidural – this is a lower-dose injection that gives pain relief without taking away all feeling in the legs, so you can still move around.

When can I have some?

As soon as the pains start to become intolerable, as long as you are definitely in labour. The effects last for several hours, but you will need 'top-up' doses, which are now often self-administered via a patient-controlled analgesia (PCA). However, it's best not to let it wear off by the time you come to start pushing, as you'll be able to do so much more effectively if you're not suddenly in pain again. Epidurals have to be administered by an anaesthetist, so you may have to wait if he or she is busy elsewhere in the hospital – women have been known to wait so long that it's too late. In some hospitals, you might not get one at all if it's the middle of the night. You won't be able to have one at home or in a birthing centre.

Is it any good?

Very effective indeed, usually – in theory, you shouldn't feel a thing once it's kicked in. Occasionally it may not work completely, and you might feel some sensation, which happened to me. I actually found that this worked in my favour as it meant I was still aware that contractions were happening. I felt this was quite reassuring, for some reason ... until it wore off completely and they came back in full force!

6The epidural was the most amazing thing. I suddenly felt human again in an instant. I sat up, had a cup of tea, had a little nap. Then it was time to push my baby out. Epidurals rock!9

Liz

What are the drawbacks?

You can end up numb to your toes, and that means you can't get up and walk around. An epidural can weaken contractions and the lack of sensation can make it harder to push: you're slightly more likely to need a forceps or ventouse delivery (see below). You'll need a drip in your arm, as a precaution in case your blood pressure drops and you need to be given fluid urgently. Your baby will also need to be monitored continuously. You're likely to have a catheter too (a tube going into your bladder, to remove wee), as you can't feel whether your bladder is full or not, all of which means your mobility will be restricted and your birth won't be able to be as 'active'. Sometimes there can be side effects, such as a fever, shaking, headache or backache.

ALTERNATIVE METHODS OF PAIN RELIEF

You don't have to be a hippy earth mother type to take a look at natural, alternative methods of pain relief. These techniques, particularly water birth and hypnobirthing, are usually welcomed into the mainstream labour ward nowadays, so if you decide to 'go alternative' in the delivery room, you'll probably find you've got support.

Lots of women find one of the following – or several, used in conjunction – helpful in the early stages of labour. And a small number will even manage to get through the whole thing on nothing more than positive thought and a back rub.

Keep an open mind – you may think aromatherapy massage will see you through 24 hours of hard labour but find, when you get to it, that only an epidural will do.

Water

Sinking into a birthing pool full of warm water is widely reported to be a very effective method of natural pain relief. It's available in many maternity units and is becoming an increasingly popular choice. Women who've used it with success say that water can aid comfort and relaxation, and often claim it helped them towards a 'calm' and 'peaceful' experience. However, once in the water, you won't be able to have any other pain relief apart from gas and air – you'll have to get out if you want something stronger.

According to the most recent figures, about 30% of women plan to use water as pain relief. A 2009 review concluded that being in water reduced the perception of pain and the need for pain-relieving drugs, but other studies suggest that, if you get into the water too soon, you can actually slow your labour down, and the likelihood of you begging for an epidural further down the line is increased. So, the jury is out somewhat – like anything to do with birth, there are no guarantees.

Acupuncture

This ancient Chinese therapy involves the insertion of fine needles into various points of the body, which, it's said, stimulates the energy channels and releases endorphins, the body's natural painkilling hormones. As with most alternative therapies, there's no real scientific evidence in its favour, and many doctors are sceptical. If you decide it could be for you, find a qualified private practitioner through the British Acupuncture Council.

Aromatherapy

Based around the power of a multitude of different natural 'essential' oils, aromatherapy is supposed to have wide-ranging, positive effects on the mind and body. These oils can be administered in a variety of ways, for example with massage, or through inhalation from a burner or vaporiser, or drops of oil infused on a hankie. Some oils are more suitable than others for labour, so do consult a trained aromatherapist for advice – or at least do some careful homework. It's unlikely that aromatherapy in itself will do very much to boost your pain threshold. But it may well aid relaxation and therefore help you cope better in the early part of labour – and it might just take the edge off the unpleasant hospital smell in the delivery room. (Essential oils shouldn't be put directly in the pool if you're having a water birth, though.)

Reflexology

This alternative therapy involves massaging particular points of the feet and is said to work in a similar way to acupuncture, by tapping into the body's energy channels and helping to release naturally occurring painkillers and reduce anxiety. Again, find a qualified practitioner to help you.

Hypnobirthing

Hypnobirthing is based on the theory that fear causes tension and tension makes pain worse, and involves putting the mind into a deep state of relaxation. To learn the techniques, you'll need to find a registered therapist – and put in lots of practice before the birth. There are also CDs available to practise hypnobirthing at home if you choose not to take a course. Anything that can get you in the zone for your birth – calm, centred and focused – will work.

I spoke to mum-of-two hypnobirthing goddess Zoe Donkin, who trained as a hypnobirthing practitioner after having had a traumatic first-time birth that ended in an emergency caesarean. Second time round she managed a calm home birth despite heavy pressure from consultants to be in hospital as her first birth was a section. Not for everyone, perhaps, but a full reversal of fortunes – and it clearly highlights how you *do* have the power to try to change your destiny if you can harness enough courage to go for what you want. These are her top tips.

- Hypnobirthing cannot guarantee the perfect birth, but it will help you have a positive pregnancy and birth. It is simply about helping women feel empowered whatever their situation. If circumstances change (baby becomes distressed and your natural birth turns into emergency caesarean, for instance) then choices must change. The worst thing is for any mum to feel like a failure.

- Hypnobirthing is a process of letting go – the opposite of cramming for an exam! Letting go of anxieties and negative expectations about birth, letting go of tension. We are also so surrounded by terrible depictions of birth in the media, we need to replace our negative connotations with more positive ones. Positive birth stories and videos are everywhere, but you need to look out for them.

- Three simple things make a big difference: breathing, visualisations and positivity. Birth shouldn't be about trying to remember lots of techniques; it should be about letting the brain shut off so your body can take over and do what it's meant to do.

- The techniques help couples relax during pregnancy and birth but are also invaluable after the baby is born … things like staying calm during breastfeeding, breathing through moments when your baby just won't stop crying, even just being mindful of your state helps (for example, my shoulders are tense, I need to breathe).

If you're interested in learning more, I've included some websites in the Useful Contacts section at the end of the book.

Breathing techniques

Slow, rhythmic, deep breathing can help you relax during labour and you're more likely to cope with pain if you relax into it, rather than tense up. Breathing can also help you conserve your energy, and boost oxygen supplies to you and your baby.

- One recommended exercise is to focus on a two-syllable word, for instance 'relax', and to repeat it in your mind in time to your breathing – 'reeeeee' as you breathe in, and 'laaax' as you breathe out. (You can use any word, but relax seems a good option.)

- Another tip is to be able to fully release tension in your face by releasing the muscles of your jaw and lips on the out breath. Try a 'sssshhhhhhh' sound, and blowing your lips out as if you're cold: 'ppprrrrrrrr'.

- You could also try counting while you breathe – or, more simply, breathing in through your nose and long and slow out through your mouth.

- Trying to keep your shoulders loose and relaxed can help reduce tension, too.

- Your birth partner can get involved and help by breathing along with you.

Massage

Just like acupuncture and reflexology, massage is said to work by putting pressure on the body's energy channels and forcing out those endorphins. And massage just boosts relaxation and well-being generally – especially when applied with a bit of love and commitment from a willing birth partner. He (or she) could try gently rubbing your shoulders, to help reduce tension, or they could focus on the lower back, where the pain of contractions is often most intense. Ask him to use long, slow, rhythmic and fairly firm strokes or circles with his fingers, or the palm of his hands – you can let him know what feels good. He may also need to bear in mind, though, that some women find that they can't bear being touched in labour, and would rather be left to get on with their contractions alone. You might need to explain this in advance to him, to avoid any offence when you tell him you will punch his lights out if he doesn't take his effing hands off you immediately.

YOUR BIRTH PARTNER

Who's the person who will hold your hand and wipe your brow while you labour to bring your child into the world?

Usually, it will be your other half, if you have one. But not everyone wants to take their man into the labour room with them and not every man is keen to go. You may prefer to take a close female friend or relative with you. In fact, research shows that this might not be such a bad idea, as you're more likely to have a natural birth with another woman in the room with you. Some women have two birth partners. You're unlikely to be allowed more than that in a maternity unit – although if you're having a home birth, there's nothing stopping you from making a party of it, should you want to. Another option available these days is hiring some professional help in the form of a 'doula' – these are trained birth assistants who offer practical and emotional support. If you're interested, find out more at https://doula.org.uk.

Whoever you choose, it's a good idea if your birth partner knows what to expect. It can be hard persuading a man to pick up a birth manual, but they need to know at least roughly what they're letting themselves in for, because if they don't, they may have a shock coming. Equally, if you're booked in for a C-section (or even if you're not, but just as a precaution), he should also have a good idea of what this will involve.

He may decide early on that he's going to stay away from the 'business end' – and maybe you're keen for him to because you're scared it will put him off the sight of your nether regions for life. Of course, one or both of you may well change your minds about this. After all, it's a pretty amazing experience seeing your kid come into the world.

To help him in his quest for knowledge, get him the hilarious but very informative book *Pregnancy for Men*, by Mark Woods (White Ladder, 2010). Or, alternatively, thrust this book at him and ask him to read the following list. It gives some ideas for useful roles a birth partner can play. (I've used 'he' throughout, for convenience.)

What your birth partner can do in advance of the birth

- Be sure he knows where the maternity unit phone number is – he might need to call them for you if you're bent double by contractions.

- Take responsibility for the journey to hospital by making sure the car's shipshape and full of petrol, and that he knows exactly how to get there (lots of people do a 'dummy run' beforehand, timing how long it takes on average) and where to park (bringing enough change for parking).

- Make sure your bag is put in the car (many a birth bag has been left behind in the commotion …).

- Have a clear idea of what your hopes are for labour and birth. You might not be in a fit state to be assertive about your desires when it comes to it. (A word of warning, though: make it clear that *you'll* be making all the ultimate decisions in the labour room. The last thing you want is a 'helpful' husband reminding you of your plans to avoid an epidural, when you've decided you really, *really* need one, after all.)

- If you're having your baby at home, it could be his job to order your birthing pool and, when it arrives, to be the person who assembles or inflates it.

THE PROFESSIONALS

What you can expect from the midwifery and maternity services available to you when you give birth will vary hugely according to where you're having your baby. And, of course, attitudes and abilities differ widely between individuals.

The majority of midwives and obstetricians are kind and able professionals who will want to help you have the best birth possible. But, as with any service occupation, there will inevitably be some who disappoint – the difference is that, while it doesn't matter that much if your hairdresser or plumber turns out to be dodgy or deficient, it's a big deal if the person who's delivering your baby does.

It comes down to pot luck, really. Unless you're having a home birth or are receiving your pregnancy care from a community midwife group, you may not have a choice about who attends you on the day itself. Nor is there much you can do about it if your labour happens to stretch across more than one shift and you're faced with a change of midwife halfway through. This can be off-putting – and downright annoying if you were getting on fine with whoever was helping you in the first place. Then again, it can go in your favour. 'I had two midwives during my baby's birth. The first was awful; our relationship probably not helped by the fact that I kicked her when she did an internal exam,' says *Modern Mum* Sara of her experience. 'However, the second was fantastic. She let me do my own thing and really helped me towards the end.'

One thing to be said, though, is that while the care you get during the birth of your baby will be influenced by what sort of midwife you get on the day, and how much pressure the unit is under, your own attitude (and your birth partner's) will also make a difference – as *Modern Mum* Melanie found. 'I ended up arguing with the midwife because I wanted to have an epidural and she was trying to persuade me not to,' she recalls. 'She was one of those "mother earth" types and was obviously not impressed that I wanted one. But I persisted, and finally got my wish.' So, like Melanie, do be prepared to speak up, ask questions and assert yourself if necessary.

BIRTH BY PLANNED CAESAREAN SECTION

You may find out in advance of your due date that you're going to have a caesarean section (C-section). This could happen if your consultant has identified a medical need during your pregnancy and thinks it will be safer for you, your baby, or both of you, if you give birth through a surgical procedure rather than in the normal way. It'll be known as a 'planned' or 'elective' caesarean (rather than an emergency one – there's more about those on page 224). Whether planned or not, caesareans are relatively common: they account for around 25% of births in this country.

There's a number of reasons why an obstetrician may want to pencil in a C-section for a first-time birth.

- If your baby is in a breech (bottom first) or transverse (sideways) position and attempts to turn him round have failed (see page 200). (Although it is possible to have a breech baby vaginally.)

- If you're expecting twins or more, since there are more likely to be complications (although in some cases it is quite possible to give birth to twins in the natural way. Any more than two babies, though, and you'll be very strongly advised to go with a C-section). For more, see below.

- If you have placenta praevia (see page 15) – in other words, the placenta is partially or completely blocking the exit of the womb.

- If you have an infection – for instance genital herpes – that could be passed to the baby during a vaginal birth.

'At 35 weeks the midwife discovered the baby was breech, so I was booked in for a scheduled C-section. The decision was really taken out of my hands and for that reason I was okay with it – I quite liked the fact that I knew the date when the baby would be born.'

Melissa

The C-section rate is currently running at approximately one in four births in the UK. Some people think that too many C-sections are carried out these days by scalpel-happy doctors who are cutting up women without good reason. Generally, however, a consultant who's keen to book you in for a C-section will have the health and safety of you and your baby at heart. He or she must consult you and explain their reasoning, and outline any risks and benefits – they certainly can't make any decision without your consent. If a C-section has been advised and you want to be certain there are no other options, you could always do a bit of your own research before signing the form.

There are also certain advantages to an elective C-section: you know exactly when your baby will arrive so can plan accordingly; the birth itself will be less painful (although your recovery won't); and, unlike the average 'normal' delivery, you'll know what's going to happen on the day.

Doctors won't automatically carry out a caesarean section without good reason (at least, not unless you're 'too posh to push', and prepared to pay handsomely to avoid doing so). However, a small number of women who have an otherwise normal and healthy pregnancy and nothing in their physical health to bar a natural birth would rather their baby was born surgically – usually due to a phobia of vaginal birth and its consequences.

Medical factfile: tokophobia

Tokophobia – an extreme fear of giving birth – was only recently identified as a medical condition and is thought to affect as many as one in seven women. If you suffer from tokophobia, counselling or some other treatment such as hypnotherapy may help you to overcome it. But if you are truly traumatised by the thought of a vaginal birth, then you should certainly relay your fears to your doctor: you should get whatever psychological support you need and, if your fears are genuine and serious, a birth by elective C-section if it's what you want.

One thing's certain: physically speaking, a caesarean section is by no means the easy option. Statistically, they carry an increased risk of complications, including abdominal pain, bladder injury, excess bleeding, infection such as endometritis (inflammation of the membrane lining of the uterus), urine infection, chest infection, wound infection, a blood clot developing, a need for further surgery, readmission to hospital and various problems with future pregnancies (although plenty of women who have a caesarean go on to have subsequent babies naturally).

You will have to stay in hospital for 36 hours or more after the surgery and recovery times are longer. If you have laboured before your caesarean, you may also be more at risk of suffering from birth trauma, a form of post-traumatic stress disorder that can, in a small number of women, kick in after childbirth. There's more on caesareans on page 224.

Risks and benefits of caesarean birth

If there are no complications and your health is good, a vaginal birth is safer than a caesarean, and also safer in terms of your future fertility. But a caesarean section is a very common and safe operation. And if you end up with an emergency caesarean, be reassured that it was no doubt the best thing for you and your baby's health.

Risks

- Babies born by caesarean are slightly more likely to suffer from breathing issues. This may be because their lungs aren't 'squeezed' out in the birth canal and so there may be fluid inside. It's usually not serious though.

- There is a small chance of the baby being cut during the operation, and some evidence that he may be more likely to develop health problems in later life.

- There is more risk of you contracting an infection post-caesarean, although this is a risk of any surgery, so is true for births with intervention as well (forceps, episiotomy).

- The healing time is generally longer than for a straightforward vaginal birth.

- There may be pain for a long time afterwards in your scar area.

- There is a risk of developing adhesions as the wound heals, which cause long-term pain and may affect your becoming pregnant again.

Benefits

- Depending on if or how much you laboured first, there will be little or no trauma to your pelvic floor (except from your baby bouncing on it for nine months) and there is statistically far less risk of prolapse, where your uterus slips down into your vagina.

- If you haven't laboured at all, you get to skip the delights of contractions entirely.

- There are no specific benefits to your baby from a caesarean birth unless the reasons for your section are to avoid a complicated vaginal delivery, where she may become stuck or distressed.

MULTIPLE BIRTHS

It's quite possible for twins to be born without a C-section – and around half are.

Your chances of having twins vaginally depends on a number of factors. Their position is probably most relevant – if the 'first' twin is in a head-down position, or both of them are, then you should be able to have a normal delivery (assuming there are no other problems, such as a low-lying placenta – see page 15). Of course, as with normal babies, twins can move around in the womb and change position, so this is a situation that you might be able to have reassessed closer to your due date. Occasionally, in a vaginal twin birth, the first baby is born in the normal way but the second has to come out via a C-section, perhaps because he's in the wrong position or an emergency situation arises.

Twins are usually born slightly earlier than most, at around 37 weeks, because there's less room in the womb for them to move around, which means they're smaller on average than singleton babies and therefore a bit more vulnerable.

When twins are born, there'll usually be more people present in the delivery room – as well as an obstetrician and a midwife, there's likely to be one or two paediatricians (doctors who specialise in the care of babies and children), just in case.

PREMATURE BIRTH

If your baby is born before 37 weeks, his birth is considered premature – about one baby in every 10 makes their appearance before this point.

ʻI didn't make it far into my third trimester as my son made an appearance six weeks early. I felt a little cheated as I didn't get to that "heave yourself around" stage.ʼ

Bella

There are many reasons why your baby might be born early, either because you've gone into labour spontaneously or because your doctor has induced you or carried out a C-section because he feels it would be risky not to. Twins or more are likely to make an earlier than normal exit, since it becomes rather a squeeze when you're sharing a womb in the late stages; and a mum's age can be relevant, with older women of 35-plus slightly more at risk of premature birth.

Premature rupture of the membranes (in other words, your waters breaking early) is a common cause, and this can be triggered by a number of things, including infection or excess amniotic fluid. Often, there'll be warning signs that premature birth is a likelihood and a midwife or doctor will pick up on these during your routine antenatal checks. One in three premature babies are delivered by C-section, because of an increased risk of complications.

Babies who are born before they're full-term can have health problems because they haven't had the chance to develop fully. They may have difficulty feeding, breathing and regulating their own body temperature. They're also more prone to infection and other problems such as jaundice or anaemia.

The good news is that special care babies, even those born quite some weeks before they're due, have a good chance of survival these days because the care and equipment available in special care baby units are so advanced. Recent figures show that babies born as early as 23 weeks have a 20% chance of survival, while at 25 weeks they have a 67% chance of survival. By 32 weeks, almost all babies will survive without any major health problems.

Modern Mum Bella went into labour at 34 weeks when her waters broke. 'Oh my God, I was a wreck', she says. 'My hormones were unbelievable – a total roller coaster. Because my son was in hospital in neonatal, and I'd been discharged, it was like the weirdest job ever. My husband and I would go to the hospital every morning and spend the day sitting with him, later learning to breastfeed, etc. And then we'd go home and have a glass of wine. Meanwhile I was expressing around the clock with the hospital's industrial machine so felt just like a cow. I cried and cried and cried. I felt like a total failure because of the bizarre birth experience. Looking back, it still makes me feel emotional now, but as with all things baby related, it passed, and gradually got better and better.'

If you go into labour early, you may be given an injection that can temporarily halt contractions, giving you time to get to the nearest unit with specialist facilities for premature babies, and for doctors to treat your unborn baby's lungs with steroids, which can help to mature them.

If you're bleeding, having contractions, your waters have broken or are leaking, or you are in any way concerned that you've gone into labour early, you should contact your midwife immediately, or – if you're really worried – call an ambulance or go straight to your maternity unit.

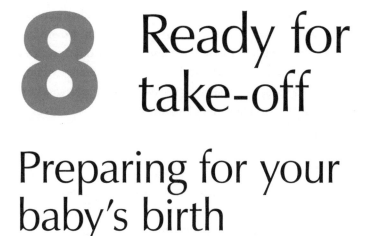

8 Ready for take-off

Preparing for your baby's birth

THE WAITING GAME

Once you leave the second trimester behind you, the novelty of pregnancy often wears off. You've ceased to wallow in the glow of people's congratulations, satisfied your cravings for Magnums, and find it hard to believe you face a further 12 weeks of growth. Round about now, most women start to find it's all become a bit of a waiting game, with birth the ultimate goal at the end of it, and a host of new or worsening physical symptoms to fend off in the meantime. For some, it can reach proportions of downright misery. Your mind can go into overdrive as the birth looms nearer. Fortunately, there's loads to take your mind off it all, as you busily prepare for your baby's arrival.

'Too much is made of having everything ready for when your baby arrives. Shops are still open if you don't have everything!'

Ele

Check-ups in the last trimester

Prepare yourself for yet more clinic visits, as you'll have more antenatal checks in your final trimester – it varies according to area, but in theory you should be seen at 28, 31, 34, 36, 38 and 40 weeks. Your midwife should always measure your abdomen, to make sure your baby's growing at roughly the expected rate (if she's worried he's not, she may refer you for a scan). And, from about 36 weeks, she'll probably have a good feel each time, to find out which way the baby is 'presenting', or lying. You'll also continue to have routine testing of your urine and blood pressure.

Labour lessons

If you've signed up for some (and you'll need to do so well in advance as they get booked up quickly – see page 21), your antenatal classes will usually begin somewhere between six and 12 weeks before your due date.

If you haven't bothered, or you didn't get a place on an antenatal course, don't fret: there's so much good information available for mums-to-be these days in books and magazines, or online, it's perfectly possible to do your own research.

Most new mums (and it's not compulsory – some are happy to go it alone) find that knowing and being in touch with at least one other woman in the same situation is a vital aid to sanity in the weeks and months after birth (and a bit further down the line, it also gives you someone to escape to the pub with). So if you're not signed up to classes and you're worried about missing out on the social aspect, then you might want to try to make a few more friends in advance of the birth, perhaps by logging onto an online community.

HOW YOU'RE GOING TO FEED YOUR BABY

Before we go on it's important to note that I personally don't have an opinion on how you should feed your baby, as I'm of the belief that we mothers must stick together in one supportive tribe, not fussing about what anyone else is doing to get through their day. It's completely up to you. But it's definitely a good idea to ponder in advance what you're going to do. The vast majority of modern mums, according to the results of the

Infant Feeding Survey of 2010, give breastfeeding a go at the start of their baby's life, and numbers are up by 5% from the previous survey in 2005. By six months, that number is down to only a third of mums still breastfeeding. You'll no doubt hear lots about how breastfeeding represents the best nutritional start you can give a baby in life, for a variety of reasons. Remember the most important thing is that your baby is fed and content and that you are a sane, happy mum, full stop. See the boxes on pages 184 and 187 for the pros and cons of both breastfeeding and bottle feeding.

At the end of the day, it's your decision and you shouldn't feel pressured either way. As with your plans for birth, it's wise to keep an open mind.

Breastfeeding

Breastfeeding, when it works, is the simplest and easiest thing. It has so many benefits for you and for your baby that it's worth considering even if just for the first few days of your baby's life. Remember that breastfeeding is fantastic for any length of time. The first creamy milk, or colostrum, that you produce is nutrient-packed, tailor-made especially for your little one at exactly the right temperature, helping to protect your tiny bub from infections.

Pressure from certain quarters can make successful breastfeeding seem like the holy grail of early motherhood. Unfortunately, many new mums simply aren't prepared for the fact that breastfeeding can be bloody hard work to start with, or that there are lots of obstacles that can get in the way of breastfeeding being established, such as tongue tie, mastitis or low milk supply (see below). If you know you want to breastfeed it will help if you can look ahead with a positive attitude. Try to be realistic in your expectations – it will take steely determination and practice to get the hang of it and make it work. If you're able to overcome the obstacles, it does get easy, I promise. It may feel like going into battle for the first month or so, but then it can be plain sailing. Soon you'll be feeding your baby while making dinner, drinking a glass of prosecco and answering the door, all at the same time. Turn to page 241 for more on the realities of breastfeeding.

'If you really want to breastfeed and there is no breastfeeding clinic nearby, I would recommend finding a good lactation consultant prior to the birth and booking her in to help you a day after you leave hospital.'

Melissa

Breastfeeding: pros and cons

Pros

- Breastfeeding is natural, therefore your milk will give your baby exactly the right nutrients, hormones and infection-busting antibodies that he needs.

- It's free.

- It's always on tap, with no sterilising, preparation or heating of bottles to worry about.

- You don't have to go to a cold kitchen to prepare night feeds.

- It may help to postpone the onset, or reduce the severity of, allergic conditions such as eczema.

- It's easily digested, making it less likely your baby will suffer from constipation or colic.

- It's a wonderful way of connecting with your baby.

- It gives you a good excuse to sit down for long stretches, watching box sets and snuggling your newborn.

- It's good for you – research shows it may help you reduce your chances of developing breast cancer and osteoporosis. And it helps your uterus to shrink down to its original size.

- It should help you lose weight, because the extra fat laid down in pregnancy is used to make breastmilk … although you do have to eat a lot of cake and sit on the sofa a lot when breastfeeding, so this point is potentially cancelled out after the first few weeks.

Cons

- The baby will probably need to spend more time feeding since breast milk takes less time to digest than formula so they don't remain 'full' as long. But it's important to remember that babies' tummies are tiny initially and they will need to feed often in the first few weeks regardless.

- Only you can breastfeed the baby, so you can't delegate the job in the middle of the night or go out for a period of time since no-one else can feed him.

- You may feel uncomfortable breastfeeding in public.

- It can be difficult, frustrating, painful and stressful to get the hang of breastfeeding.

Preparing to breastfeed

You'll need to be practically (as well as mentally) prepared for breastfeeding. Have the following ready.

- **Breast pads** – leaking is just one of the joys. It's temporary, while your breasts adjust to your baby's demands, but you can get through dozens in the early weeks. One thing to be prepared for is that, while your bub is suckling at one boob, the other will start to leak milk. I found this to my cost when I was wearing a new light grey nursing top but had forgotten to put on a breast pad. Baby was happily feeding away on one boob, and on the other side I had an ever-expanding dark wet patch growing on my top. Nice!

- **Nipple cream.** Sore nipples are par for the course, so have a tube of nipple cream on standby – midwives usually recommend Lansinoh, which is made from a pure form of lanolin.

- **Breastfeeding bras.** It's a good idea to have at least three or four. As with other areas of maternity fashion, underwear has now been updated and there are some lovely ranges of pretty and comfy nursing bras out there.

- A selection of **tops** that either lift easily or unfasten down the front. Lots of high street shops now offer nursing clothing and you can't even tell they're designed for breastfeeding. And scarves will be your friend as they offer a handy shield or distraction if you want to cover your boob when feeding out and about. Really though, it's possible to feed your baby and no-one be any the wiser around you – not a hint of flashing mammaries. Wear a vest, with a top over it. Top comes up, vest pulls down, boob's your uncle. Because you're not flashing any flesh (and baby's head covers your nipple when he's feeding), it really is discreet and spares you blushes. Although you might find you simply don't care very much. I'm sure half of London has seen my boob by now and I haven't really noticed.

- **Muslins** are a real boon when breastfeeding as they mop up spills, and can be draped over your shoulder and chest to provide a little privacy.

- A **breast pump** will be useful a bit later down the line if you want to express your milk into a bottle so someone else can feed your baby. (However, to allow yourself a good chance to get breastfeeding established, don't try this for the first four to six weeks unless you're advised to as a way of increasing your milk supply.)

'When your husband sees you pumping milk out of your massive veiny boobs you do wonder if there will ever be any sexual desire between you again!'

Natalie

There's not much you can do to prepare your nipples for the onslaught, and there's no point in either applying cream or putting yourself through the torture of 'nail brushing' them in a bid to toughen them up. Those babies will rise to the challenge when the time comes. Babies tend to feed, feed, feed for the first couple of days and nights. With my second, I remember feeling I had created some kind of nipple vampire as he was permanently attached to my boob for an entire night the third night of his life. This is evolution's way of ensuring your supply is kick-started to meet baby's demands. So, it won't last forever, but it is very sore and, needless to say, can be a bit of a shock if you're not expecting it.

There's lots more information on breastfeeding on page 241. It's a good idea to read this now so that, when the time comes, you are prepared for some of the hurdles you may have to overcome.

Bottle feeding

The alternative to breastfeeding is, of course, bottle feeding. Its main advantage is that it requires less of a physical commitment from you as your partner can share feeding duties. The reason there's not as much on bottle feeding in this section isn't a deliberate bias – there's just less fore-thought needed and, frankly, fewer challenges on the road.

Bottle feeding: pros and cons

Pros

- It's easy to learn how to bottle feed.

- Anyone can bottle feed the baby.

- Father and baby get more chance to bond as he can take his turn bottle feeding.

- You don't have to worry about what you're eating (or drinking!) passing through to your baby.

Cons

- Formula doesn't have the same infection-fighting antibodies as breast milk.

- You have to get up in the night to sort out and warm the bottle.

- You need to spend time cleaning and sterilising, which can be a lot of work. If you travel, all this stuff has to go with you.

- Making up bottles can become a rather tedious chore.

- You have to pay for formula.

Preparing to bottle feed

It's not difficult preparing bottles, although it's highly tedious, and the process can become somewhat soul-destroying when you make up your 16th that week. Cleanliness is everything so don't be tempted to cut corners, and be prepared for a rigorous routine. Follow the manufacturers' instructions carefully, and make sure you get the quantities right. You will need:

- some **means of sterilising** bottles, lids, teats and formula scoops. A steam steriliser is the quickest and easiest method

- **bottles, teats and lids**

- **formula.** Make sure you get the right age range – you want the one for newborns, not 'hungry baby', which could cause them to be seriously constipated, or 'follow-on-milk' (which most health visitors will tell you is an unnecessary bit of marketing, anyway).

There's more on how to bottle feed on page 249.

SHOPPING NECESSITIES

So, what do you need? At this stage, the answer is 'not much'. Parents-to-be are often superstitious about getting equipped for their baby too early, and the fact is that you don't actually need more than a few basics to start out with. Most people also find that they get lots of clothes (often beautiful, but somewhat impractical) as gifts. And you can always go shopping a bit later – online, if not in person.

On the other hand, you really do need to get your freshly discharged offspring something to wear, something to sleep on, and something to transport him in. And it makes sense to get the basics in with plenty of time to spare, just in case of a premature arrival. Your baby's basic needs at the start are as follows.

- Up to 10 **vests** and the same number of **sleepsuits** (get the sort with enclosed feet and you won't have to worry about keeping a pair of socks on him). Newborns really don't need any other sort of outfit: they want something comfortable, and you want something you can get on and off them easily (which you'll need to do very frequently, since milky vomit and green poo stains abound).

- **A cardigan** for colder weather (perhaps two so you've always got one clean).

- **A pramsuit or snowsuit**, unless it's a very warm time of year.

- **A hat** (ditto).

- Lots of teeny-tiny **nappies** – way more than you probably imagine. Newborns need their nappies changed a *lot* – at least every couple of hours or so, 24/7, for the first week. Disposables are the most convenient, but if the environment's a concern for you, and you can face the laundry issues, you could think about reusables. You'll also need a job lot of cotton wool and some barrier or nappy cream.

- **Somewhere to sleep:** a cot or Moses basket. The basket is nice because it's cosier for a tiny baby and you can move it from room to room, which, since they sleep so much when they're tiny, is very useful. However, they only fit in them for three to five months, tops, and so they're not very economical. Most people borrow one – but for safety reasons, it's recommended that you always buy a new mattress. (There's more information on safe sleeping on page 267.) You can get 'co-sleeping' cots that attach to the side of your bed, for the first six months of your baby's life. I had one and they're a godsend, particularly if you've had a C-section, as it means, if you're breastfeeding, you don't have to get up and down so much to feed your baby overnight – baby is right there next to you but safely in his own space.

- **Bedding.** Get the fitted variety, and buy quite a few as they can get a lot of milky vom on them. You'll need one to two, depending on the time of year, lightweight blankets – the cellular sort, with holes in, are ideal. Some people swear by baby sleeping bags as baby can't chuck them off and, provided you get the right size, are suitable from birth.

- **Muslins.** The must-have accessory for mums. Once the baby's born you'll probably be walking around with one permanently draped over your shoulder, to mop up the many and varied messes that are about to feature in your life.

- **A car seat.** You won't be allowed to leave hospital (assuming you're going home in a car) without one of these. Buy new or, if you're taking on one that's second-hand, only accept from a good friend, in case it's been damaged in an accident, which could compromise its effectiveness.

- **A pram and/or sling.** The pram market's a huge one, and it's a pretty big purchase, so take your time and definitely, definitely try before you buy. Buying second-hand on eBay is great for saving money but prams really do need a test drive as they're so much a part of your daily life. (I spent many a month bitterly regretting the monster three-in-one model we invested in without much thought – it required a degree in engineering to put it up or down, and was so heavy I could barely lift it into the car boot.) Features to look for are how light or sturdy it is; how well it 'handles'; how easily it can be collapsed and put up; and whether you've got enough room to store it at home. Slings are a popular option as they're less of a faff and less space-consuming than prams. They can also be useful if you need to get something done around the house, but your crabby baby refuses to be put down. Slings are also an absolute godsend for soothing fussy babies through kangaroo care, keeping them close to your heart.

- **Something to wash him in.** You'll probably just 'top and tail' (see page 263) for a couple of weeks, anyway, and even then, a baby bath isn't really necessary as you can just use a large, clean washing up bowl until he's a little older and can be safely held in the big bath. However, a baby bath on a stand, or one that fits over the main bath, is a godsend if you have a bad back. Baby toiletries really aren't necessary for a newborn – in fact, their delicate skin could well do without them.

COPING STRATEGIES FOR THE FINAL STRAIGHT

You really don't need to paint the skirting boards. I say that because, in actual fact, I really *did* paint all the skirting boards in our house while on maternity leave with my first baby. And I'm still not sure why. So, with the benefit of hindsight, could I insist you resist the urge, if possible, to take on any major DIY or cleaning projects in the run-up to your baby's birth? Lots of women get a surge of energy in late pregnancy and feel compelled to remove dust from unseen corners and get a new coat of paint on the walls as they await their baby's arrival, usually put down to the so-called 'nesting' instinct, but quite often because they're simply bored out of their minds during maternity leave.

Modern Mum Charlotte decided to give in to the urge of building decking in her garden while 39 weeks pregnant … and at the end of a full day of decking, baby Frances made her appearance.

Whether or not it's a real biological imperative, there's no doubt that it's tempting to try to get the house in order, because you won't have a chance once junior's your main priority. However, the real truth of it is that your baby won't actually give a toss what her immediate environment's like and, as you'll have more important stuff to worry about and really do need to conserve every ounce of energy you've got for the physical challenges ahead, you'd do well to take the same attitude.

For fairly obvious hygiene reasons, a clean(ish) kitchen is a good idea (especially if you're bottle feeding), and it's useful to clear all floor surfaces of any tripping hazards. But really, major renovations and decorations during pregnancy are a waste of time. It's true you won't have much time to sort the house out after the birth, but then again, once your baby grows into a toddler, there'll be even less point, since he'll wreck it in any case.

As for the nursery, make it look beautiful if it pleases you to do so. But otherwise, content yourself in the knowledge that your baby will probably be in with you for a while and, even once you've moved him into his own room, many years will pass before he takes any interest in interior design (if at all).

Things to do before your baby is born

- Have a good old tidy up, but don't obsess about a designer nursery.

- Do a big shop of basics such as loo roll and staple foods, so you don't have to worry about shopping once you've brought your baby home. Make meals for the freezer, if you're that way inclined. But bear in mind that all the big supermarkets deliver – so if you don't get a chance or you can't be bothered to stock up, you're unlikely to starve.

- Get some sleep, a bit more sleep, and yet more sleep. You're not going to get a good night's kip for months (and possibly years) to come.

- Do some research into birth and think about how you hope yours might pan out (see page 158).

- Read up on baby care. Lots of new mums realise they were so busy reading about pregnancy and birth, they forgot to work out how to look after their baby. As they say – they don't come with instructions.

- Go out – for a meal, to the cinema. When your baby is born, your social life will go on a bit of a hiatus and morph into something slightly different – coffee dates with other new sleep-deprived mums rather than cocktail nights in heels.

- Go for a 'babymoon' with your partner. Whether a proper holiday or a relaxing mini-break, it's a great idea to get away with your other half for a while – preferably with plenty of time to spare in the pregnancy, so you don't have to worry about going into labour in a strange place (and bearing in mind that most airlines won't let you travel late in pregnancy). Some travel companies are actually marketing 'babymoons' now, and there's also a growing number of hotels and spas that offer what's described as a 'complete antenatal package'.

- Get your legs and bikini line waxed and your nails, face and/or hair done. Okay, so it's not compulsory, but some women find it makes a huge difference to their state of mind. Book into a salon for professional help where necessary, though – you attempt to wax your own bikini line at your peril. They say it's a good idea to have your hair cut into an 'easy to maintain' style, since organising to go to the hairdressers once your baby is born becomes slightly more tricky and tends not to be top of your list.

- Practise some relaxation and breathing techniques, and some birthing positions. It's true that this may make you feel slightly foolish, but it could help when the time comes – and, hey, it's passing the time, isn't it? If you're hoping your birth partner will be on hand with a bit of pain-relieving massage, get him (or her) to have a trial run – without the pain, it will probably be quite enjoyable.

- Pack your hospital bag. It's a good idea to have this by the door ready to go at least a couple of weeks before your due date. (Try to put it somewhere you won't fall over it, though.)

Growing pains

Late pregnancy can be a time of much physical misery. You may well find some of your 'niggles' get worse, or that you get a whole new set.

- **Exhaustion.** Just lugging around all that extra weight is enough to make you tired. That's before you take into account the insomnia (see below). Don't do too much.

- **Discomfort.** Fully expect your entire posture to change towards the end of your pregnancy. If you've ever seen a woman clearly nearing the end point of gestation, tummy thrust out and legs splayed as she walks – or rather, waddles – you'll already have a good general idea of how your gait is likely to change. Your balance may also be affected, too.

- **Breathing difficulties.** As your womb expands, it puts pressure on the lungs, making it harder to breathe. There's not much you can do about it, but rest and take it easy whenever you get the chance.

- **Backache and pelvic pain.** This tends to increase in later stages as the added weight puts pressure on your spine and forces you into a curved posture. Try to rest, do some regular, gentle ab-strengthening exercises, stick to sensible shoes, and watch your posture.

- **Tummy pains.** As the ligaments stretch to support your growing uterus, it's normal to feel some pain and strain in your tummy area, although it can be a bit worrying if you're not sure what it is. Chat to your midwife – she'll almost certainly be able to put your mind at rest. You may also begin to experience Braxton Hicks (see page 203), or practice contractions, which feel like a tightening sensation across the tummy – in fact, these occur throughout pregnancy, but aren't usually obvious until the third trimester. Although generally passed off as 'painless', some women report that they're pretty uncomfortable towards the end.

- **Rib pain.** Caused by the womb pressing against the ribs, and also sometimes by your baby, bless his little football boots, attempting to bend it like Beckham inside you.

- **Leaky boobs.** Your breasts may leak a little colostrum – the golden, nutrient-rich precursor to ordinary breast milk – during the third trimester. If it's bad, you'll just have to crack open the breast pads.

- **Indigestion and heartburn.** These can happen because your digestive organs are being thoroughly squashed by the lack of space. It may also affect your appetite. Try cold milk or Gaviscon.

- **Insomnia.** An increasingly active baby and difficulty in trying to find a single remotely comfortable position mean that getting a good night's sleep gets harder the nearer to your due date you get. There's only one way to get any comfort in bed in the late stages, and that's lying on your side, so inevitably you can start to yearn for a different position. And also, of course, you'll have lots on your mind as you dwell on what lies ahead. (Round about now you might begin to start having some seriously weird dreams about birth and your baby. It's normal.) Pillows will help – in particular, you'll find that one placed under your bump and one in between your knees can provide some relief.

- **Itchy tummy.** As your skin stretches over your growing bump, the result can be itchiness and irritation. A non-perfumed emollient, such as aqueous cream, or some calamine lotion, might help. But don't forget that extreme itching in the third trimester can be a symptom of obstetric cholestasis (see page 52), so keep an eye on it.

- **Swollen feet and hands.** Medically known as oedema, it's normal for water retention to worsen in this phase of pregnancy. However, it's also linked to pre-eclampsia (see page 41), so it's a good idea to keep your midwife informed. Try to rest and put your legs up when you can.

Anyone for perineal massage?

Your perineum (in case you don't know) is the area between the vagina and anus, and during birth it inevitably comes in for a right old battering, very often tearing as the baby's head comes out. Some people reckon you can help to avoid this by using your fingers and a little oil to massage the area daily in the last three to four weeks of pregnancy – there's a specific technique, which your midwife can show you. Word of advice: the word 'massage' makes it sound like a pleasant experience. It's not. Essentially, you are preparing the area to be stretched during childbirth, stretching it by degrees, more every time. It is apparently very effective at preparing the area's ability to stretch to make room for your baby's head and makes it less likely for you to tear during birth, emulating the 'burning' feeling of your baby crowning. I did all the perineal massage but ended up having an emergency caesarean, so I can't personally vouch for its efficacy, but I can confirm that it burns and it's slightly faffy to do with a massive bump. If you do try it, make sure your hands are clean and your nails short, and choose a lubricant that won't irritate – wheatgerm oil is said to be the best (it's available from health food shops: if the assistant smirks, she knows what you want it for). One of the main problems in trying to massage your perineum is access: a huge bump can make this somewhat challenging. If so, you'll have to ask your partner to do it for you. (And this is where you find out just how much he loves you …) You can also buy a balloon that inflates inside you for the same purpose of stretching the perineum. *Modern Mum* Jo said this was brilliant and definitely helped her recognise when she was dilating in labour. There are details in the Useful Contacts section at the back of the book.

Raspberry leaf

Taking a regular dose of this herbal remedy in the last six to eight weeks before your baby's birth is reckoned to help tone the uterus and encourage a shorter labour by making the contractions more effective. There's no scientific evidence to back this view, but some women swear by it. You can take it in one of two forms: either in a tablet or by infusing the dried leaves in hot water to make a tea – both are available from health food shops. Don't take raspberry leaf tea any earlier in pregnancy, though.

PACKING YOUR BAG

You'll need to get together a bag for your hospital stay and keep it by the door, at least a couple of weeks before your due date. Assuming things go without any complications, you probably won't stay in hospital for longer than a day and the night afterwards.

Even if your visit turns out to be short, you're going to need a certain amount of stuff to see you through labour and birth – plus things for however long you hang around for afterwards. In fact, by the time you've got what you need together, you may find it fills three bags: one for labour, one for afterwards, and one for your baby. If you end up with so much luggage it's causing a blockage in your hallway, streamline it to just the essentials.

Stuff to pack for you

- **Something to give birth in.** Although most hospitals will provide a gown, you might feel more comfortable in something of your own. Make sure it's something you're happy to throw away afterwards, which you will almost certainly want to do once it's covered in blood, sweat and afterbirth – an old, baggy t-shirt is ideal. Taking two is probably a sensible precaution, in case you need to change midway through.

- **Maternity towels.** These are not the same as ordinary sanitary towels – oh no, they're bigger and more absorbent – so make sure you get the right ones for the job. You may also get through rather more than you imagined – so stock up with several boxes, and take at least one to hospital in case you have to stay a while.

- **Big pants.** You'll need some super-sized knickers to fit your big sanitary towels in. Buy a cheap multi-pack of new ones – you'll get good use out of them for a few weeks after the birth, after which you can chuck them. Take at least six pairs, as you'll probably be changing them frequently.

- **Nursing bra and breast pads.** Try to get measured for a bra as near to your due date as possible – but bear in mind you might also need one in a size up, as your boobs will get even bigger when your milk comes, two to three days after the birth (see page 255).

- **Bottles and formula.** For bottle feeders, it's best to be prepared with your own equipment as hospitals increasingly are focusing on breast-feeding and not offering formula, although in practice they will always be able to feed your baby if you're completely underprepared. You can buy formula starter kits from Boots – these have a number of ready-prepared feeds and are perfect for the hospital stay. At home you'll need a good supply of formula, plus steriliser and bottles.

- **Front-opening nightwear.** You'll want something nicer to slip into once you've taken off your blood- and amniotic fluid-soaked t-shirt, and a front-opener's ideal for breastfeeding.

- **Comfy clothing to change into before leaving.** You'll still be flabby, and every bit of you will ache. A loose, soft tracksuit should be just the job. Don't make the mistake of assuming you'll fit into pre-preg wear suddenly, as you might not. Maternity waistline is best.

- **Toothbrush and toothpaste, and some basic toiletries.** There probably won't be anything in the hospital and one thing you're almost certain to want afterwards is a shower. So take shower gel or soap, and shampoo.

- **Hairbrush and make-up.** It may sound shallow, but you will want to take pictures of you and your baby in hospital and not look too horrendous. Or you could just Instagram filter it …

- **Warm socks and/or slippers.** Hospital floors can be pretty cold. Some women also like to keep socks on during labour. (These can also end up covered in gunk, so, again, make sure it's a pair you're not attached to.)

- **Snacks and drinks.** Catering can be a hit-and-miss affair in maternity units, especially if you become hungry or thirsty in the middle of the night, so bring your own sustenance. You might feel hungry during labour – and you'll very likely be ravenous afterwards. Have something non-perishable in your suitcase, like crackers or cereal bars, and pop in fresh stuff like fruit just before you leave. Don't forget some cartons of juice or bottles of water too. Top tip: keep cartons of Ribena in the freezer, then on D-day chuck them in your bag – they'll stay really cold for the hours of your labour and provide sugary refreshment when you need it.

- **Boredom busters.** Labour can be a long drawn-out affair and, frankly, it can get tedious (especially with an epidural in place!). Take a good book, some magazines, an iPad or lots of things to watch downloaded onto your phone to help keep boredom at bay.

- **A camera.** This is one photo opportunity you won't want to miss.

- **Your phone.** You'll want to text everyone you know with the news once the baby's born, and put in a call to any loved ones. Remember that hospitals generally have rules about turning mobiles off, though. You may also want to make sure you've got change for a payphone in case you can't get a signal.

- **Lip balm.** If you're planning on having gas and air, this is essential as you may get dry and cracked lips.

- **Sponge; water spray; stereo or your delivery music of choice.** All optional extras.

'I couldn't believe how much time I'd spent worrying about what to bring and then didn't really need any of it. Especially worrying about what I would wear for labour and birth ... I was apparently quite happy to strip off!'

Julie

'Bring your own pillow in a favourite pillowcase – it'll be much more comfy and makes you feel like you're at home – and a flannel.'

Hannah

Stuff to pack for the baby

You won't need to take much to the hospital for your baby, other than several soft cotton sleepsuits and vests; a cardigan or jacket; a hat (depending on the weather); a blanket for the journey home; nappies; and cotton wool.

Most important of all is the car seat: unless you're walking home, the hospital won't let you leave without one of these.

THE THINGS PEOPLE SAY

The bigger you become, and the closer to your due date you get, the more annoying the comments you can expect from other people. It's human nature to be fascinated by the sight of a woman's body as it carries out the awe-inspiring role it was designed for. So try to be understanding when people want to give your belly a little stroke, or ask: 'Haven't you had that baby yet?' And hard though it may be, you must resist the urge to throw back a sarcastic reply like: 'Yes I have. The baby's at home and now I'm just really fat.'

If the touching bothers you, just ask them politely to refrain. As for stupid observations ('My goodness, you're that big and you still have four weeks to go?') and 'helpful' birth advice ('You'll be fine! I managed on gas and air alone'), try to take it with good grace. If you can't do that, just ignore them.

YOUR FEELINGS

Make no mistake, the final weeks of pregnancy can be a pretty hard-going time emotionally, too. It's normal to feel utterly fed up with your condition and absolutely desperate to get your baby out. It's also quite usual to be terrified about what's ahead of you – and not just birth, which, let's face it, is at least over within a day or two. Parenthood, on the other hand, is something you'll have to contend with indefinitely. Now *that's* scary.

Aim to take your mind off your fears by filling your final baby-free weeks with stuff you won't be able to do soon and concentrating on all the positives – in a very short time, there'll be a third, rather adorable (if needy) small person in the house. You might find a bit of relief from some gentle exercise helps you to relax. And you should try to spend some quality time with your other half, talking through any worries with him. He's probably scared, too, and could do with the reassurance himself.

Reading up on birth is important, because you need to be prepared, but equally you don't want to get too obsessed with what's ahead and become panic-stricken. What will be will be. Try thinking about something completely different sometimes. See friends, or take in a good movie – whatever you did to enjoy yourself before the alien invasion (other than boozing).

YOUR BABY'S POSITION

From around 28 weeks, your midwife will start feeling your belly to check his position. By now, the majority of babies will have turned round to a cephalic, or head-down, position, ready for birth, but some will be 'presenting' bottom or feet first (breech), and occasionally a baby will lie in a transverse position (sideways). Often, a breech or transverse baby will move round of his own accord in time for birth and, if not, he can sometimes be encouraged to wiggle round.

You can also try to coax your baby round yourself. One trick is to lie on your back close to a wall, placing your feet high up against the wall, and then, using the wall for support, lift your hips as high as you can. You can cushion your back, shoulders and hips with pillows. Try to spend 15 minutes doing this three times a day. You could also try spending as much time as possible on all fours and wiggling your hips. Just don't try this in public.

It's not unusual for a baby who's turned to flip back again. And if your baby remains steadfastly in the breech position by the time he drops down into the pelvis ready for birth (as an estimated 3% do), your consultant is very likely to advise a planned caesarean section. However, it could still be possible for a breech baby to be born in the normal way if you're keen to give it a try, and there are no other complications. A persistent transverse position can signal other potential problems, though, such as a placenta praevia (see page 15), and so if your baby's determinedly taking a sideways view of life by the very end stage of pregnancy, you'll inevitably have to undergo further investigation and prepare for the likelihood of a C-section.

Most babies with their head down will be in what's known as the anterior position as you approach your due date – in other words, with the back of his head facing your front. However, some end up the other way round, with the back of the head towards the spine. This can cause severe backache during late pregnancy and birth. Neither way matters at this stage though. Due to the shape of our pelvis, he has to look sideways to be able to get his head into it, and only then, when labour is well advanced does he need to turn – hopefully so that he is looking behind you, with the back of his head at the front.

Engagement

For a first baby, at some point from around 37 weeks, and sometimes earlier, your baby's head will 'engage'. In other words, the little monster drops down into your pelvis in readiness for birth. (This process is also sometimes known as 'lightening'.) It can give your lungs and ribs relief, but may give your bladder and pelvis some grief instead. You can't win 'em all.

Your *absolutely* final checklist

Okay, so are you ready for this? Don't forget the following.

- Pack your bag – and your birth plan, if you have one.
- Have your maternity notes ready to take, if you've been keeping them at home.
- Make sure the house is reasonably shipshape and you've got a bit of food in the freezer.
- Keep the car in working order and full of fuel.
- Put your birth partner/person responsible for transporting you to hospital on red alert (hint: they'll need to stay sober so they can drive at short notice, and they need to always be at the other end of their phone).
- Have numbers for your midwife or maternity unit in a prominent place.
- Have a car seat and the few basics your baby will need ready.
- De-fuzz your legs and bikini line. A girl's got to have some dignity, after all.

---

9 Labour day(s)

What happens when you give birth

So, here we are. You thought the piles and the back pain were bad, well, this is the bit that really hurts (usually). It may be easier said than done, but please don't get too scared at the thought of labour. Yes it hurts, yes it can go on for a bloody long time, and yes it can often turn out to be a bit more complicated than you might hope for. But with a tiny, tiny minority of exceptions, births in this country almost always work out all right in the end.

You can't know what having a baby's like until you've actually had yours. But you can get a rough idea of what's coming and prepare yourself to some degree simply by having a good old read of the following chapter. I've tried to be as honest as possible. And I've gone with the stance that it's better to know what will or could happen than to be unprepared and then wonder WTF's going on when the time comes.

'I wish I'd known that for the most part labour is fundamentally boring. It is tedious, monotonous, relentless and ruthlessly boring. It requires incredible stamina of the brain to continue to believe that at the end of the process you'll have a baby.'

Nicki

YOU'RE NEARLY THERE …

Your body may start to gear itself up for labour a few days or even weeks before it actually kicks off. So although they can be useful indicators that the time's approaching, there'll usually be no need to panic at the onset of any of the following signs. Give the maternity unit a quick call if you're worried – the duty midwife will probably tell you to make a cup of tea, put your feet up, and wait for your baby in as relaxed a way as possible.

What to look out for

- An increase in or thickening of **vaginal discharge**. It's normal to have some throughout pregnancy, but towards the end it can increase, caused by the baby's head pressing on the cervix.

- **Backache**, or a period pain-like feeling.

- A 'show'. This is when the jelly-like plug (it looks like heavy discharge and will often be streaked with blood, which can be a little alarming) that seals the cervix comes away. It can do this some days or even a couple of weeks in advance of labour beginning, or it may not happen until the last minute.

- Stronger **Braxton Hicks**. These 'practice' contractions actually occur for a long time before your due date – it's just that they don't always become noticeable until later and can become really quite intense, and uncomfortable even, in the final few weeks. Lots of first-timers wonder if the Braxton Hicks they're experiencing are real contractions. (If you're not sure they're strong enough to be real, the truth is that they probably aren't.)

- A bout of **diarrhoea**. This can happen sometimes in the 24 hours before things kick off, as Mother Nature clears out the bowels in readiness for labour.

GOING PAST YOUR DUE DATE

It's not particularly unusual for an EDD to come and go without so much of a hint of your waters breaking or contractions starting. Normal pregnancies can continue for up to 43 weeks – and due dates are only an estimate, remember.

Going past your due date can be an anti-climax, and a considerable strain when you feel your tummy's already at bursting point. My first baby hung on in there for two weeks beyond his expected birth-day, so I know the suspense can be crippling. Although frustrating, it's nothing to be alarmed about. However, your maternity team will be keeping a careful eye on you because, in pregnancies that go beyond 41 weeks, the risk of a baby being stillborn or becoming distressed starts to rise slightly.

If there's no sign of your baby by your due date, you'll usually be offered a 'membrane sweep' before anything else is suggested – your midwife or doctor will run a finger round the inner edge of your cervix to encourage it to start dilating. It can be uncomfortable, or actually really painful, and may make you bleed a bit, and it can also cause cramps, so if you're booked in for one, don't have anything else planned for the rest of the day.

If this doesn't work, you'll usually be offered a day in the next week to have your labour induced – in other words, to get things going by artificial means. Most doctors will be keen for this to happen within 14 days of your due date but it will depend on your hospital's policy. It could even be 10 days – even if your pregnancy has been normal and there are no other risk factors. They should explain why they want to induce and what the risks and benefits could be. But you should still be offered the chance to wait for labour to start naturally if you prefer. If you do choose to wait, your doctor will probably want to see you frequently – possibly daily – to check that your baby's doing okay.

It's very normal to hope to avoid induction – it could mean a very abrupt and intense start to labour pains (for which you may need to consider some heavy-duty pain relief, such as an epidural). You don't have to have an induction if you don't want one (your labour will start at some point – it has to!), but your doctor will usually only recommend induction if he's concerned about you or your baby. For example, once your due date has passed, you are less likely to have a stillbirth if induced and less likely to deliver by caesarean than if you wait beyond 42 weeks for natural labour. A common misconception is that you go into hospital to be induced and bingo – your baby is there within a few hours. Sadly, although this is possible, many inductions go on for a couple of days before they kick-start labour. Although the most common reason for induction is a simple matter of being overdue, other possible reasons for it include the following.

- Your baby's growth has slowed or stopped, suggesting that your placenta has stopped working efficiently, or it is coming away, which could affect the oxygen supply to your baby.

- Your waters have broken and there's an increased risk of infection.

- You have an existing medical condition such as diabetes or heart disease, or a pregnancy condition such as pre-eclampsia or gestational diabetes, and your doctor thinks your baby (or you) would be safer out than in.

There's more about induction on page 214.

Natural ways to encourage labour

Rumour has it you *might* be able to put a rocket under your baby's arrival with the following methods. The only evidence that any of them work is anecdotal rather than scientific. Still, you've nothing to lose (and, in some cases, a fair bit of fun to be had) in trying. Steer clear of these altogether if you've had any complications, and don't wear yourself out by becoming obsessed.

- **A hot curry.** If eating spicy food really does work as a way to bring on labour, then it's probably something to do with a laxative effect that stimulates the uterus as well as the bowel. There's no scientific evidence whatsoever that it works, but still, as you might not get to go out for a curry for a while once your baby's born, you may as well get one in while you can. Don't attempt to have a really hot one if you're not used to it – this isn't the time for a stomach upset.

- **Hot sex.** It's unlikely this in itself will bring on labour, although the theory is based in scientific evidence, since seminal fluid contains prostaglandins, which are said to soften the cervix, and the hormone oxytocin – which stimulates contractions – is released when a woman orgasms. You shouldn't have sex once your waters have broken, because of the risk of infection.

- **Nipple stimulation.** This aids the release of oxytocin, same as when you orgasm. The idea is to use your palm and rub both nipple and areola (the dark skin surrounding the nipple) in a circular motion. You need to be pretty committed, since it's reckoned that you need to do this for an hour three times a day if it's actually going to work. (That's a lot of tweaking.)

- **Pineapple.** This tropical fruit contains the enzyme bromelain, which is said to boost the production of prostaglandins. You'd have to eat it in large quantities to get enough of the stuff to be effective, and by then you're probably looking at the same sort of effect as a hot curry.

- **Raspberry leaf tea.** Although this might be helpful in preparing the uterus for birth if taken in the last month or two of pregnancy (but no earlier), it's a myth that a single dose or cup will trigger labour.

- **Reflexology, aromatherapy, homeopathy and acupuncture.** Practitioners of all these alternative therapies claim they might give a natural kick-start to labour. There's no science to back those claims, but they might be worth a try if you've got an open mind. Contact a qualified practitioner first – and be prepared to pay.

- **Long walks or walking up and down stairs.** Moving around and keeping upright could help for the simple reason that gravity might jiggle your baby further down towards your cervix. Take a stroll if you're up to it, but don't try anything too strenuous at this point – you need to save your energy.

WHAT HAPPENS WHEN YOUR WATERS BREAK

At some point, the sac of amniotic fluid surrounding your baby will burst and spurt or dribble out from your vagina – this is commonly known as your waters breaking. For most women, this doesn't happen until after contractions have begun and labour has started (and sometimes they're popped for you by a doctor or midwife as part of an induction process – although you don't have to have your waters broken for you, and you must pipe up if that's something you want to avoid). If you're really lucky, your baby might stay cocooned in her little sac for the entire birth and come out peacefully still surrounded by cushioning amniotic fluid.

'My waters breaking felt like a really big wee that I couldn't stop. He was breech, which was why it was such a dramatic torrent!'

Bella

For about one in 20 women, waters break before labour starts. So if your waters go but your contractions haven't yet begun, it's a sure sign that they soon will. You should give your midwife a call if it happens to you. You'll probably be asked to go in for an assessment because, once your waters go, there's an increased risk of an infection travelling up your vagina and reaching your baby.

You might be offered an induction at this point, or given the option to take a 'wait and see' approach, in which case you'll be sent home but asked to be vigilant for possible signs of an infection, such as a high temperature or changes to the colour and smell of your amniotic fluid. In nine out of 10 cases, labour starts within 24 hours of waters breaking early. If it goes beyond that, an induction will probably be recommended as the infection risk will continue to increase.

It's a bit of a cliché, but it's true that your waters can break without any warning, which might cause a slight embarrassment if you're in public. 'Mine went while sitting on a friend's mum's white sofa,' confesses *Modern Mum* Katie. 'Thankfully she was lovely about it.'

Although the experience can sometimes feel like a huge, watery gush, it's not as much as you imagine – and some women find it amounts to no more than a trickle. The fluid should be very pale in colour or clear, sometimes with a little blood, or a pinky tinge. If there's any green or brown in it, or if it is very bloody, call the maternity unit straight away to let them know. They'll probably want you to go in for an assessment, as this could signal a potential problem.

HOW MUCH DOES IT HURT?

The start of proper contractions means the first stage of labour is definitely underway. Contractions – also known as labour pains – are what happen when the muscles of the uterus flex as it works to open up the cervix (the neck of the womb), from where your baby will soon be making his exit. They're almost always mild to start with (you may even mistake them for Braxton Hicks) and spaced far apart – perhaps every 20 minutes. This stage, known as the latent phase, can go on for ages – a whole day or even two is not unusual, particularly in a first birth.

Overall, it's hard to say how long a first-time labour's likely to be, as it varies so much, but between 12 and 24 hours is usually cited as average (with many of the *Modern Mums* reporting labours longer still than that).

‘It's a very surreal feeling giving birth – I felt like a train wreck but also superhuman.’

Caroline

It's a good idea to stay upright and active if it happens during the day, and to try to sleep or doze if it's night-time. Try to have something to eat and drink, too, if you can, to boost your strength – although admittedly some women do feel off their food around now (and sometimes nausea or vomiting occurs). This is also a good time to have a bath, to help you relax – it may also soothe the pain of the contractions. Other ways to pass the time in as relaxing a way as possible include going for a gentle walk, watching something you love on telly, listening to your favourite music, or getting your other half to give you a massage. A good tip for coping with the milder pain of early labour is to pop a couple of paracetamol, which should take the edge off a bit.

'I remember telling my unborn child I was very sorry she would never have a sibling as I was never ever going to do this again. In the final throes of labour I felt incredibly animal and basically roared my baby out of my body. I needed throat lozenges the next day as I had been growling so hard.'

Nicki

What do contractions feel like?

It's really hard to describe what contractions feel like, as they can vary so much from one woman to another. Some liken them to intense period cramps; others say they are far, far more painful than that. Some women feel them in their abdomen, others in their back. And some women find they are really quite bearable, even without any pain relief, while others are shocked at just how agonising they are. I personally felt that contractions were completely manageable with breathing and visualisation ... until I had been in labour for over 24 hours and I had my waters broken. Then immediately, with one particular contraction, it became an avalanche of pain that rocked my body and I found I didn't have a chance to breathe through them. I began to feel very panicky that I couldn't cope if they got any worse than that one epic tsunami of a contraction that took over my body. At that point I demanded an epidural ...

I have had many more accounts from ladies who went into labour naturally of how contraction pains felt completely manageable as they built up to a crescendo gradually, so with each one you're more prepared for the next and it's like riding the crest of a wave – get the breathing right and you'll sail along with it until the end; miss the timing slightly and it might crash over you. Most importantly, remember that with each contraction, you are that little step closer to meeting your baby, and all that pain will be a distant memory. There's a reason we can go on happily to have more children. Amnesia.

Descriptions from the *Modern Mums* vary.

- 'A searing horrendous pain.' (Liz)

- 'Like someone jabbing you with a knife.' (Manna)

- 'Almost like your body was being held in a vice and the grip becoming tighter and tighter.' (Kat)

- 'It was all in my arse and cramping like I just needed to do the biggest poo.' (Nicola)

And if all that sounds scary, take comfort in the thoughts of these *Modern Mums*.

- 'It felt like the baby was just moving around vigorously – no pain at all.' (Bella)

- 'Like a bad period pain.' (Maria)

- 'A bikini wax is much, much worse.' (Rowan)

- 'It felt like my back was really hurting – it wasn't in my belly at all.' (Naomi)

- 'It was intense, but I felt completely normal in between each one – it totally disappeared.' (Jess)

So there you go – I told you it was variable. One thing most women do agree on, though, is that if you relax rather than tense up through contractions, you'll be able to cope with them better.

Things that could be a worry in early labour

There's no need to go into hospital or even call the maternity unit during early labour if your contractions are well spaced and you're coping. However, you should call your midwife straight away in the following cases:

- You're bleeding heavily, although a certain amount of blood as part of your 'show' is normal.

- Your waters have broken and are stained with a green/brown substance – this is likely to be meconium (your baby's poo) and could indicate that he's in distress, or be a sign of an infection.

- You have a pain in your tummy that's constant (as opposed to coming and going, which is what contractions do).

- You have a sudden or severe headache or vision disturbances, which could be a sign of dangerously high blood pressure.

- You don't think your baby is moving any more, or your baby seems to be moving around in a frenzy.

WHAT IF MY BABY WON'T WAIT?

As most first-time labours last at least a day or two, you should have loads of time to work out if you're actually about to have your baby before heading to the maternity unit (and still have oodles more time to spare when you get there). Once in a while, though, a first-time mum can be taken by surprise with a very short labour and a baby who arrives before she's even had time to pick up the telephone. If it happens to you, here's what to do.

- Try to call someone who can be with you quickly, if you don't have anyone there already.

- Ring the emergency number on your notes. They'll make sure someone comes to you. If you can't find the number, dial 999 and ask for an ambulance. Make sure the front door's open so they can all get in.

- Try to find some towels – one to save your carpet, and a large clean one to wrap your baby in.

- Kneel with your head on your forearms and keep your bottom as high up in the air as possible. Resist pushing if you can. Try breathing in a pattern of three short pants and a long blow. This can help delay things a bit.

- If you can't resist the urge to push and your baby starts to make its way out before anyone's got to you, don't panic. Hold on to him, and carefully check to make sure the cord isn't looped round his neck (ease it gently back over the head if it is, but don't pull it).

- Once your baby's all the way out, wrap him up to keep him warm. There might be mucus or fluids in his nose preventing him from breathing properly, which you can push out by stroking down the sides of his nose.

- Place the baby on his front across your belly with his head lower than his body to allow any remaining fluid to drain out, and firmly rub his back with the towel.

- Don't attempt to cut the cord – the professional who comes to your aid will sort that for you – but do cuddle him close and try putting him to your breast. Your placenta should follow soon afterwards, still attached to the cord.

'ESTABLISHED' LABOUR

Eventually the contractions will begin to come more often, be longer-lasting, and feel more intense. Once they're coming thick and fast – every four to five minutes, say – you're considered to be in 'established' labour.

Even now, you're very likely to be between six and 12 hours away from having your baby. Generally, midwives encourage you to stay at home for as long as you can before coming in to hospital, assuming there are no problems and that you're coping with the pain. After all, if you've got to hang around waiting, you may as well do so in the comfort of your own home.

Make a call to the unit once your contractions are coming regularly, every five to six minutes or so. You could then be advised by the duty midwife to come in (especially if your waters have broken by then), or you may be advised to stay put a while. If you do go in, and the midwife establishes that you've still got a long way to go, you might be sent home again.

IN HOSPITAL

If you've been advised to go in, or you turn up anyway, a midwife will take your pulse, temperature and blood pressure and check your urine. She'll feel your abdomen to check the baby's position, and listen to the baby's heartbeat. Then she'll probably carry out an internal examination on you to see how things are going: as labour progresses, the cervix gradually dilates (opens up), and when the midwife examines you she's checking to see how far along this process has got. If she says you're '1 centimetre dilated', then you're only just at the start. Labour isn't considered to be 'established' until the cervix is 3–4cm dilated, and you're not 'fully dilated' and ready to go until it opens up to 10cm. You might get sent home if you are not in established labour – which can be heartbreaking when you feel you need some proper pain relief immediately – and told to come back when your contractions are closer together or last longer.

Until you're coming close to the moment of pushing your baby, your midwife will probably leave you and your birth partner to pass the time together in the delivery room. She'll pop in from time to time to check you're okay, to listen to the baby's heart rate, and to see if you're any closer to being fully dilated. Meanwhile, move around if you can and put your breathing and massage techniques to use to help you cope with the pain of contractions. But pipe up if, at any point, you're not coping with the pain and you need something to help you. There should be a button you can press to alert your midwife.

Electronic monitoring

Usually the midwife will keep a close check on your baby's heartbeat during labour with a hand-held monitor. But in some cases – if your pregnancy or labour is considered high risk for some reason, or a complication has arisen – she may want to wire you up to a piece of equipment called an electronic fetal heart rate monitor. This works by using two sensors attached to a machine that straps onto your belly with elastic belts, and that can read your baby's heartbeat and your contractions. From this, your midwife or doctor can get a printout of this information in the form of a graph, and they can use it to see how your baby's coping during the labour.

Although reassuring and painless, the drawbacks to electronic monitoring are that it makes moving around and changing position difficult and it can make you feel like the subject of a science experiment. You might be more comfortable sitting in a chair while you're being monitored, rather than lying on a bed.

BEING INDUCED

About one in five women in this country end up having their labours artificially induced. If an induction is suggested, you should be given a full explanation as to why, and of the risks, benefits and alternatives, and given time to think about and discuss it before making a decision. You should then be told about the different ways in which your labour might be given a helping hand.

There's no set way for an induction to proceed – it could make things happen very quickly; you could end up waiting for many hours (or even a couple of days) for action; and, in some cases, it may not work at all (after which the usual route will be caesarean section – this can be pretty demoralising news if you've already spent an exhausting couple of days on the induction trail).

What does induction involve?

The first attempt at inducing labour will usually involve you having prostaglandin. This is a synthetic version of the very same hormone that's released naturally in labour (and, yes, from semen) to soften the cervix. This can be given in the form of a tablet, pessary or gel that's inserted into the vagina. One dose may not work, and sometimes a second or even third dose will have to be given. And it's quite possible it won't work at all. If it does, you've had a result, because it's a gentler method than what comes next and, in theory, your contractions shouldn't be any stronger than they would be in normal labour.

If nothing happens (usual in about half of cases), your midwife or doctor may attempt to speed things up further by breaking your waters. This is done by inserting a small hook-like instrument into the vagina and making a small tear in the membranes – it's not supposed to hurt but may cause you some discomfort.

If this doesn't work, you'll be offered the next stage – Syntocinon (which is the artificial form of oxytocin, the natural hormone that triggers contractions), given via a drip into a vein in your hand or arm. So, all in all, your ability to move around will be very restricted. A drip has other major disadvantages, too – it can cause rapid and very strong contractions (so you may well need an epidural to cope with them) and it can put your baby under stress, so your baby will need continuous electronic monitoring.

HOW YOU MIGHT ACT IN LABOUR

Keeping active and upright can make labour easier as gravity is working for you, trying to encourage baby to press down on your cervix. So walking around, bouncing on a birthing ball, getting down on all fours and wiggling your hips from side to side, or draping yourself in different ways over chairs, beanbags or mats could all help you find a bit of comfort and relief from the pain. You won't need to feel self-conscious about doing any of these things, even if you do suspect you look like a mad woman in the process – the staff will have seen it all before.

The position that you actually give birth in is said to make a big difference, too. Lots of women find crouching on all fours, or kneeling, squatting or standing with support from a birth partner, are more comfortable and natural stances. And it makes sense when you think about it, because of the helping hand from gravity.

If you feel strongly that you'd like to be free to move around or to experiment with different positions, write this in your birth plan.

EFFING AND BLINDING

There's a time and a place for everything, and the delivery room is not the place for social niceties. Fact is, you may find yourself acting in a less-than-sedate way during labour. Different women respond in different ways, but the truth is, it's such an extraordinary experience that you'll more than likely surprise yourself with some fairly extraordinary behaviour. 'I never, ever swear normally, but with every contraction, I was shouting 'fuuuuuuuuck' at the top of my voice,' says Sarah. 'I was at home for quite a lot of my labour – so I did offer apologies to the neighbours afterwards!'

It's very common to let rip whatever extremes of emotion you're feeling on whoever's in the room with you. Midwives won't usually take it personally if you're rude to them – they're pretty well used to it – but you should perhaps point this out to your birth partner *before* the big day, so he's psyched up for the possibility of being insulted or even assaulted. There was a point in my labour overnight when my husband was having a nap on a mat on the floor and I actually kicked him during one contraction and told him to 'fucking wake up!!' Sorry, my love, it wasn't me it was the contraction. You may feel a need to transfer your pain, which is potentially bad news for your birth partner. A few *Modern Mums* told me of holding their partner in a headlock. Beware of digging your nails in so hard it draws blood …

Whatever surprising things you do in the throes of labour, you don't have to feel embarrassed about it. (And, you know, you probably won't. In fact, you probably won't give a flying *fuuuuuuuuuuck!*)

> ## What your birth partner can do for you during labour and delivery
>
> - Keep you entertained (or just provide company) if you're enduring a long, boring wait for action.
>
> - Massage your back to help ease the pain.
>
> - Fetch you snacks, drinks or anything else you need.
>
> - Help keep you cool by sponging or spraying your face.
>
> - Offer words of encouragement and support.
>
> - Speak up or ask questions if something's happening you're not keen on or sure about (but only if you give them the nod first …).
>
> - Provide support if you want to give birth kneeling, squatting or standing up.
>
> - Let you know all's going well from his vantage point down 'the business end'.
>
> - Keep a low profile and his mouth shut if you need him to!

HERE COMES YOUR BABY

In between the first and second stages of labour there sometimes comes a brief phase known as 'transition'. Contractions are incredibly intense and coming thick and fast, and you may feel shaky or sick, confused, distressed, and at the end of your endurance. It means you're close to the end, though, and you're about to enter the second stage of labour: pushing out your baby.

As your baby's head moves right down through the cervix towards the vagina, you might feel a very intense pressure in your bum – almost as though you need an almighty poo. And you'll probably experience an overwhelming urge to push (you might hear this referred to as 'bearing down'), but if it's not yet time to do so, because the cervix isn't fully dilated, your midwife will ask you to hold back. You can help counter the urge to push by breathing in short puffs or pants.

'I started experiencing the natural expulsive reflex, where I could feel my body pushing my baby down. I suddenly got very excited that the end was in sight and asked my midwife if this meant I was in transition. She examined me and said I was fully dilated!'

Caroline

Pushing

When the time's right, your midwife will want you to push with each contraction, and she'll guide you in doing this. A lot of mums report that they weren't quite sure how to do the pushing, and the piece of advice on this that crops up most often is to 'push like you're doing a poo' – that is, through your bottom rather than through your fanny. Once the head begins to appear, you may want to put your hand down to feel it, or even take a look with the help of a mirror. Your midwife will urge you to stop or slow your pushing, breathing out in puffs if it helps, so she can guide the baby out slowly, which will minimise the risk of your perineum tearing. Once the baby's head is out, the hard work is done: you should only need to give one more push to get the body out.

In some births, a baby will pop out relatively quickly and easily, but in others it's a truly knackering process that can take some time – up to an hour, or sometimes longer still. If you're not comfortable at any point, get the help you need to change position.

Sometimes, in spite of your best efforts, your baby won't budge – perhaps because he's got himself into an awkward position, his head's too big to get through the birth canal, or your contractions have ceased to be strong and effective. When this happens, your doctor might suggest using forceps or vacuum extraction (ventouse) to help him out (see page 222).

How much is this going to hurt my vagina?

Unless you're still benefiting from the effects of an epidural, you'll find that pushing your baby out stings pretty considerably – hardly surprising, really, when you weigh up the size of your baby's head against the size of your vagina. However, if you've already been through a long labour and many hours of agonising contractions, the truth is you'll probably find this the easy bit.

Lots of women suffer a torn perineum while pushing their baby out. Although this sounds horrendous, the reassuring truth is that at this stage of birth you're usually so focused on (and amazed by) your baby's entry into the world that you don't really notice the pain. If the tear is a small one, it will probably be left to heal on its own. If it's deep, though, it will have to be sewn up. For more on that, see the section on episiotomy below.

Could I poo myself when I'm pushing?

This is one of those things that can cause a certain amount of advance horror among first-timers. It's only later that you will realise the truth: if you poo yourself during labour – which you might, because of all the pushing – it will be the *absolute least of your worries*. Farts and urine may also make their escape. Fear not, in any case: your midwife will be on the alert and will wipe any mess away, pronto, so you might not even notice. (And if you happen to poop yourself while in the birthing pool, you'll get to find out what that little fishing net's for …).

‘When I was pushing I vaguely smelt something that I thought might have been poo – the main thing I'd been dreading – but no-one said anything and I couldn't have cared less at the time.’

Jacqui

YOUR BABY'S OUT!

Once your baby's born, the midwife will usually put him straight onto your tummy so that you can help hold and see him. This 'skin-to-skin' contact calms your baby, promotes bonding, and helps to get breastfeeding off to a good start.

The midwife will then quickly look him over and make a speedy routine assessment of his breathing, skin colour, heart rate, muscle tone and reflex response, known as an Apgar score or test. She will wipe off some of the slimy mix of blood, amniotic fluid and vernix your baby's likely to be covered in as drying his skin stops him from getting cold, and put a dry towel or blanket over him.

Meanwhile, the umbilical cord will be clamped and cut – this is one small way in which your partner can play an active part in your baby's arrival, although, if he's squeamish, he might prefer to forgo this option. Once the placenta has been delivered, you'll also get stitches now, if you need them. You may feel as high as a kite at this point, or you may feel drained and slightly depressed. Both are normal.

Occasionally, a baby will need his air passages suctioned and sometimes a little extra oxygen, in order to help him breathe, in which case the midwife may take him to a resuscitaire, a small heated cot.

Your baby will also be offered vitamin K, either in the form of a single injection or as two or three separate oral doses; this protects against another very rare but dangerous condition, vitamin K deficiency bleeding (VKDB).

Don't be surprised if your baby looks kind of hideous. As well as being rather slimy, newborns can be hairy, blotchy, somewhat swollen, squinty-eyed and pointy-headed. Luckily, he'll be beautiful to you.

'A good friend of mine told me that however unbearable the pain is, once the baby is out it stops completely, and that was a very useful thing to keep in mind because it was absolutely true.'

Natalie

Delivery of the placenta

It's not quite over. While you're focusing on your new baby, contractions (though thankfully milder ones) will continue as your body prepares to expel the placenta, usually described as being the size of a small dinner plate, often with a little more pushing needed from you. This is the third stage of labour.

This process should happen naturally within an hour or so of the birth. If you're keen for a natural delivery of the placenta, it's something you could put in your birth plan. However, it's common these days to be given an injection to speed things up and reduce the chances of excessive bleeding, known as postpartum haemorrhage (PPH). This is known as a 'managed', rather than a natural, third stage, and involves an injection into your thigh and the midwife placing one hand on your belly and gently pulling the cord with the other to remove the placenta, usually within about 30 minutes of birth. (It may well cause you a bit more discomfort, but it won't be anything like as painful as pushing out your baby.) If you decide to let the placenta come out of its own accord and this process is prolonged, or it causes you to bleed heavily (which it might), your midwife might again suggest an injection to move things along.

Sometimes (in about 2% of births) all or part of the placenta is left behind because it's still stuck to the wall of the uterus – known as a retained placenta – and, if it's not removed, it could also lead to a haemorrhage. If this happens, the midwife will probably try giving it a tug to ease it out, but if it's still not coming you might need a small surgical procedure, known as manual removal of the placenta. For this, you'll need a local anaesthetic such as an epidural (or a top-up, if you had one for the birth anyway), and you'll be taken to an operating theatre.

You may or may not be interested in sneaking a look at your placenta – it's played a pretty important role over the last nine months, after all. Or perhaps you'll want to take it home and carry out a symbolic burial of it under a tree in your garden, something mothers in Malaysia do.

Since it's said to taste a bit like liver and contain properties that help ward off postnatal depression, you may even want to borrow a controversial recipe from TV chef Hugh Fearnley-Whittingstall and make placenta pâté from it. (Add shallots and garlic, flambé, puree, and serve on focaccia bread.) Or some people have their placenta made up into supplements to take postnatally to help build up their strength. If you do dish up placenta as a side order, my advice would be to not invite your mates.

AN ASSISTED DELIVERY

If your baby needs help to be born because he's stuck, or if you're getting too exhausted to eject him under your own steam, you may end up having an assisted birth. This means the obstetrician will use either forceps or a ventouse to get a good hold of your baby and ease him out. Forceps are curved tongs that look a bit like a large pair of salad servers. If these are used, you'll need to have an episiotomy (see below) to allow room for the forceps to fit inside you and round your baby's head. A ventouse is more like a sink plunger: it has a plastic or metal cap that fixes to your baby's head, and a vacuum pump which is used to cause a suction effect. While both of these things look and sound terrifying, it might help to bear in mind that they're pretty commonly used and your obstetrician will be experienced in wielding them.

Ventouse is more common and is the gentler option of the two as it is less likely to require an episiotomy and you're less likely to suffer any damage or pain as a consequence, but forceps are more likely if your baby is still quite high, or is distressed and needs to be born quickly. Babies born with assistance will usually bear temporary marks as a souvenir: forceps can leave red marks on the temples, while vacuum extraction can cause swelling and a misshapen head – this goes down within a few days and will have sorted itself out completely within a week or two.

In either case, you'll need to lie on your back and have your feet placed in stirrups. You'll also need pain relief in the form of a local anaesthetic or epidural. Usually, a doctor will try one of these methods, but not both. If it doesn't work, he'll then suggest a caesarean section.

There's a school of thought that intervention techniques such as these are too often carried out unnecessarily, robbing women of their chance to deliver naturally, and cause stitches, bruising and even more long-term damage to the pelvic floor or perineum that could have been avoided. The other school of thought says used at the right time by a skilled practitioner, they can improve the outcome for your baby, and can reduce the chance of pelvic floor damage or bad tearing. You're well within your rights to question your doctor's decision (or get your birth partner to do so). However, you might find that, by the time an assisted delivery is mooted, you're only too grateful for your baby to be helped out in any way possible.

EPISIOTOMY

A word every woman dreads. This is a cut of the perineum and vagina, performed by a midwife or doctor when considered necessary to help your baby make his exit. It's not as horrible as it sounds – at least at the time – as you'll be given effective pain relief in the form of a local anaesthetic injection (unless you've already got an epidural in place).

You'll need to be stitched up again afterwards (as indeed you may be if you tear naturally) and unfortunately this can cause much soreness, itching and discomfort after the birth – not to mention abject fear of having a poo (which can lead to constipation, and an ensuing vicious circle). It should take a month for the stitches to heal completely. They can become infected, though, if you're not completely vigilant about washing (after all, your priority tends to be your newborn and it's understandable that you might not get much time to shower, etc.), leading to more misery. For some women, poorly healed stitches can have consequences months down the line. An episiotomy will generally take a bit longer to heal than a natural tear, so most midwives will try to avoid it for this reason. Make sure it's in your birth plan if it's something you really, really don't want. See page 250 for more on your body after birth.

'If you've had a tear or episiotomy, use Sudocrem after a few days and it protects everything when you wee (ouch) and you can also pour a jug of warm water over your lady-bits while you're weeing. Oh, the glamour!'

Bella

IF YOU NEED AN EMERGENCY CAESAREAN

It's a good idea to know roughly what an emergency caesarean involves, just in case you end up having one. This section will tell you what you need to know, ahead of the possibility.

'I wish I'd known that you can see your reflection in the lights of an operating theatre as I am a bit haunted by the image of me, white as a sheet, being prepped for surgery.'

Bella

Sometimes in a labour that has started off normally, an obstetrician may decide that the fastest and safest way to get your baby out is by performing a caesarean. For instance, one will probably be mooted if:

- your labour isn't progressing and you're getting exhausted, or your baby is stuck.

- your baby isn't getting the oxygen he needs, or his heartbeat pattern has changed or he is becoming distressed.

- a potentially dangerous complication such as placental abruption (see page 67) has occurred.

Usually, a doctor will have a good reason for wanting to carry out an emergency C-section, and as you won't have much time to get a second opinion, research possible alternatives or even think it through, you'll have to put your faith in their judgement. However little time there is for discussion, though, your doctor must explain their reasoning, and ask for your consent. If you'd planned on a natural birth, you might feel disappointed and frightened at being whistled into surgery; reassure yourself with the knowledge that C-section is a very common surgical procedure – and that, ultimately, giving birth to a healthy baby is what matters, not how you do it.

What happens in a C-section

Once you've given consent for a caesarean to be carried out, you'll be given an anaesthetic. Usually, this will be in the form of an epidural. However, in some emergency cases you may need to have a general anaesthetic, and if this is the case, your partner won't be able to come to theatre with you. You'll also need a catheter – a tube that empties urine from your bladder – and a drip in your hand, to administer fluids or pain relief when needed.

Once the anaesthetic's kicked in, an incision is made, usually horizontally across the lower part of the abdomen at the top of the pubic bone or 'bikini line'. It's done this way so that the scar won't show from underneath your pubic hair. Very rarely, in certain emergency cases, a 'vertical' cut is made. This action all takes place behind a screen.

A second cut is then made in the uterus so the baby can be lifted out. He'll be handed straight to a paediatrician – who will have been invited along as a matter of routine – to be checked. If he's very small, or poorly, your baby will have to go straight to the special care unit. If not, he can be handed to your birth partner or carefully placed next to you or on your chest for a cuddle while you're stitched up: this is a major bit of suturing, and takes about half an hour.

If you've had a C-section, it will take you longer to recover than with a vaginal delivery. And if your C-section was an emergency, it's likely to be longer still. There's more on recovery after a C-section on page 258.

AFTER THE BIRTH

Your baby's out! Sometime soon after you've had your baby – assuming she's well and doesn't need special care – you'll both be taken to a postnatal ward where, more than likely, you'll be left to your own devices for a while. You may want to sleep, but you may still be buzzing and want to spend some time holding, or just staring at, your baby.

‘Without a doubt the most powerful moment is the moment the midwife places the baby, blood and all, on you for a cuddle. I was so shocked by this wonderful warm creature. It was the most emotional moment in my life.’

Ele

I can remember feeling quite blown away at this point after my first baby's birth, having been taken up to the post-labour ward in the dead of night. It was almost unreal – a moment I'd so often experienced in my daydreams, now come true. Typically, anxiety struck almost immediately (a feeling that hasn't really let up since) as my son was the only baby on the ward who was crying. By daybreak, I'd had about five minutes' sleep and I still hadn't quite got my head round the reality – my baby was no longer inside me, but lying next to me in a small plastic hospital cot, crying loudly.

Please don't worry if, when you've had your baby, you don't find yourself looking deep into their eyes, convinced you've never loved anything so much in your life. It doesn't always work that way, as *Modern Mum* Nina explains. ‘I never bought into that view that once you're holding your baby you forget the pain and fall in love – what a load of bollocks! I'll never forget the pain to my dying day and I couldn't possibly love someone I hadn't got to know. So, although I felt a very strong sense of responsibility and was relieved he was okay, I didn't love him. That came a little later, as we got to know each other and learned to live together.’

Fear is another very common emotion at this moment. ‘It's a combination of overwhelming love and terror,’ recounts *Modern Mum* Sara. ‘I was in a state of physical shock from the delivery, then there was the shock of actually holding my baby for the first time, and it was overwhelming. The baby I'd been trying for for three years was here, no longer a hope or a fantasy but a real, breathing being and I was thrilled by my dream coming true at last, but also terrified by the sudden responsibility. I was shaking like a leaf.’

10 Birth stories

Six *Modern Mums* recall their labour day

These six real birth stories from our *Modern Mums* are to show just how diverse people's experiences can be. Try not to ever get drawn to people's 'horror stories'. The harsh fact is that no-one can tell you or predict what your birth will be like. Always remember that your birth story is going to be unique to you and your baby. Knowledge is power, so do your homework, be prepared for anything, hope for a pinch of luck and a light sprinkling of good fortune when the time comes, and allow yourself the strength to go with whatever flow your baby needs to enter the world safely.

One of my *Modern Mums* had an emergency caesarean. When I asked her to share her birth story with me she said, 'Is it relevant as it wasn't natural?' And to that I say, *all* birth is valid, relevant and never, ever a failure. If your birth doesn't go as you 'planned', give yourself more praise for coping when things went in a different direction. However your baby comes out, you must take time to give yourself a massive pat on the back for being so bloomin' amazing and know that no man ever, not even the most powerful man in the world, can ever do something as powerful as give birth to another human. (Note to very hormonal and overly emotional readers: these stories might make you cry!)

'You need to mentally prepare yourself for childbirth, not just physically. It was the toughest thing I've ever done, from both aspects.'

Hannah

Becca's birth story

At about 2am I got up for my nightly loo trip. The previous day I had been getting mild cramp-like feelings – it was also the day after my due date so I knew baby was coming. As I wiped I got a shock of red blood. So I called the maternity unit at the hospital and they said that I should come in – they said it was probably nothing but I should get checked out. My husband was still snoring. In denial about what was most likely to be about to happen, I told him what the hospital had said and that I would get a taxi on my own. Half asleep he agreed and I got dressed in the dark. With the taxi arriving imminently, my other half changed his mind. But we left my hospital bag (read ginormous suitcase) in the bedroom.

When we got to the hospital they checked me over. They hooked me up to a machine and monitored the baby's heart rate – it was a bit fast – and it was at that moment they told us that we wouldn't be leaving hospital without our baby. I nearly vomited. Things moved very slowly – I wasn't really contracting at this point. My husband went back to the house to get the bag (and he managed to find time for a 'quick' shower). At around 9am my husband disappeared for a fry-up to keep his strength up (!) and by 12 midday the staff wanted to speed things up so the midwife broke my waters. From then all hell broke loose. My contractions sped up to every few minutes. I went from being about 3cm dilated to 10cm dilated in about three hours. Gas and air were my saviour. As my body went through the weird and odd calmness of what they call transition and the primal urge to push took over my whole body, the midwife guided me through pushing out my baby. At this point my fears about shitting myself were confirmed – but midwives really are experts at whisking it away – and, to be honest, at this point I really couldn't care less. High on gas and air, I had my husband in a headlock and at one point told him how much I loved him. My midwife gave me a snip and after a few more pushes my little boy entered the world in a whoosh and a squelchy slap onto the bed.

At first he didn't cry, and along with the massive sense of relief there was also a feeling of panic as they whipped him away and massaged his little chest out of my line of sight, leaving me asking 'Is it okay?' over and over. Suddenly there was a little gravelling squawking and a little bleating sound as his lungs found air, and as he was handed back to us, swaddled and clean, we asked what sex he was. I always had a strong feeling that he was a boy – so it wasn't really a surprise – and as I looked at him I felt totally overwhelmed about meeting the little person who had been inside me for so long. In all his squashed, wrinkly perfection. We all cried – the adrenaline and the emotion coursing through our bodies.

Jessica's birth story

We were keen to have a home birth, so we read lots to make sure it was the right decision for us. I was also lucky enough to have the support of my mum and a close family friend who agreed to be my midwife.

When we knew that things were starting to happen, my midwife Becky instructed me to take two paracetamol, have a large glass of red wine, get in the bath and then go to bed. I was up from about 2am, unable to sleep and counting the minutes between contractions on an app. At 9am Becky arrived and we started using the TENS machine, which was a great distraction as the contractions got harder. I found my best position was kneeling on cushions with my head in the sofa, but found it surreal that I could be there having a contraction one minute and then back at the table chatting the next!

As the contractions got harder I was sick a couple of times. I then felt ready to get in the pool that we'd set up in the living room. It was like getting into the best bath in the world ever. Warm and comforting and above all it really allowed me to move positions so I could get onto my knees for the contractions and lie back in between. The water carried my weight, which was fantastic as it became harder to move around as I got more tired. I went into a trance-like state in between the contractions, conserving my energy.

Just at the point when I didn't think I wanted to continue, the feeling changed and my body started to push. As I could feel the baby's head moving down I felt so calm and just listened to Becky as she slowly talked me through the last bit to make sure that I stretched to let the baby come out slowly and didn't tear. Joey caught our baby and passed her through to me. We couldn't believe it. It was just incredible.

We sat for quite a while in total amazement until we thought to look to find out we had a girl. Then in our own time we cut the cord and Joey sat on the sofa and had his first proper cuddle with his daughter. I came out of the pool and fed her for the first time, which was so much harder than I thought, but we persevered and learned together.

I genuinely really enjoyed the experience of giving birth. We did it. We had help and support but we had a normal straightforward labour in our flat and were allowed to do it our way.

Zoe's birth story

Zoe's first birth was an induction followed by an emergency caesarean. She then trained to be a hypnobirthing practitioner, and applied her hypnobirthing techniques in her second birth.

I did everything differently in the lead-up to the birth second time round. None of the endless pineapples and curries, sweeps, reflexology, acupuncture that I did before. I thought I was helping him come out, but in fact I think I was scaring him into staying inside where it was so warm and cosy. Second time round, I stayed totally relaxed, focused on my baby coming when she was ready, and believed that nature would do its work. Although the consultants tried to convince me of the risks of uterine rupture and to go into hospital, I decided to continue with my plan for a home birth. I knew I would be most relaxed at home and that I could be quickly transferred to hospital if I felt anxious or if there was anything amiss. We made our home cosy, filled it with flowers and energy snacks, and I stuck up positive affirmations.

On Saturday morning, exactly a week on from my estimated 'due date', my Braxton Hicks got stronger. I thought it might still be practice labour but I asked my sister to come and pick my son up so that my husband could stay with me. My instinct told me it was worth us bedding down at home. I lay in bed watching a funny film and eating breakfast in bed.

Soon these waves of pressure increased in intensity and frequency until I was having to breathe through them. It dawned on me that I might be in labour, even though I'd had no show and my waters hadn't broken. I asked James to ring the midwife and let her know that she needed to be at the ready but not to come just yet.

The midwife arrived 20 minutes later to find me lying on the bed still relaxing. She listened to baby's heartbeat, which was totally normal.

My birth plan said that I didn't want any unnecessary internal examinations. However, I felt it would actually be really good to know how dilated I was, because if I was only 1cm then that would be fine and just mean more relaxing without the midwife there. In fact, the midwife was surprised to find me 5cm dilated and swiftly said she would stay with me! As baby was so low down, she asked me to tell her as soon as I could feel any urge to push as I could progress quickly and she would need to get another midwife along.

The time between being 5cm dilated and feeling the need to push seemed to go in an instant. As I moved myself around on my birth ball and listened to the hypnobirthing CD, I felt calm and in control. Then this instinct to bear down took over and I found myself making some pretty primal mooing sounds as each surge came! At that point the midwife called her backup, and luckily the birth pool was finally ready.

I got in and felt an immediate sense of relief, but after around 45 minutes I started to feel too hot and baby's heart rate was going up a little. The midwives thought it would be a good idea for me to go to the loo and see if that would help move things along. It did! The surges became much more intense. My husband kept telling me how well I was doing, which really helped. I could only stand this intensity on the loo for a little while before going back to our bedroom. Here I found myself kneeling by the bed and an uncontrollable urge to push, after which my baby's head emerged.

The midwives told me that on my next surge the rest of her would probably be born. Lo and behold, her body came out and I brought her up to my chest from beneath me. Holding her warm little body against my skin was dreamlike. I felt so out of it and at the same time completely present. She cried and nuzzled and soon began to feed while I sat holding her in disbelief and awe.

There's no two ways about it, childbirth is amazing and epic. I suddenly felt tired, shaky and nauseous and it took me just over an hour to birth the placenta.

The midwives left us alone, and we found ourselves lying in bed with our new baby, unable to quite take in what had happened – that she was inside me and now she was here, and that it had all gone so smoothly. It felt like a miracle.

Nicola's birth story

At 41 weeks and five days I was taking 15 minutes to get out of bed, had had five sweeps, and I'd definitely had enough of being pregnant.

At 6pm on 7 January I went into hospital for my last chance at an outpatient induction. Vanessa, my midwife, was awesome and incredibly professional. She reassured me that I could still stay at home through the early stages of labour but once I was getting closer to giving birth I would have to return to the hospital.

At the hospital I was looked after by two lovely female staff – one doctor, one midwife – who sat me on a bed and completed the obligatory monitoring before inserting the pessary. I went home, hopeful.

Some 45 minutes after going to bed my waters popped and woke me up. Three contractions in and I was *wailing* into my pillow. Ray immediately called my midwife, Vanessa, who, upon hearing my screams in the background, ordered Ray to take me straight to the hospital. Within minutes my contractions were coming thick and fast. I screamed all the way to hospital. I was convinced that my son was going to be born on the pavement. But weirdly I felt calm and in control. Each contraction was doing something. I could feel it and I was excited – really fricking painfully excited.

We were rushed in and greeted by my lovely midwife and somehow I dealt with the pain, on my hands and knees, pressing my head into the bed. I have no idea how much time had passed when Vanessa said, in the calmest voice imaginable, that I should start pushing and not be scared. That was all I needed to hear to let rip, and now my body was doing what it was meant to and it was the single most empowering moment of my entire life. My body literally took over – it was as close to an out-of-body experience as I can relate to. At one point Vanessa asked me if I'd like to touch my baby's head as it appeared. I could feel him and it was wonderful.

Who knows how many contractions, how many minutes later, Vanessa held the Doppler to hear my baby's heartbeat, and it was way too slow. In the same voice she had used before, she simply said, 'On the next contraction we need to get your baby out, Nicola.' When that wave came I pushed with more might than I knew I possessed. I think even Vanessa may have been surprised at the speed with which my little boy was unceremoniously ejected as she called to me, 'Slow down now,' in an effort to preserve my perineum, but honestly I simultaneously thought 'How?!' At 1.55am on Thursday 8 January we welcomed our son into this world.

Jacqui's birth story

My baby was due on the Monday and I was convinced that, as it was my first, I would probably be two weeks late and probably have to be induced. On the Tuesday prior to my due date I got a bit of a show. On the Wednesday morning, I started having period pains. In the afternoon, I suddenly noticed that the period pains were starting to come and go … and they were very slowly getting slightly stronger. By late afternoon, they had turned into definite contractions, although they were still very (*very*) mild. I went to bed and the mild contractions continued all night. I did manage to sleep, but it was very broken and I was quite anxious as I'd expected the baby to come in the night.

On Thursday morning, the contractions pretty much stopped, so my husband went to work. By the afternoon, they came back again but this time they were definite contractions and I sometimes found I had to stop talking or walking to focus on the contraction. I put the TENS machine on and found it quite useful, but more as a distraction. I walked down to my local shop to get some paracetamol and was furious because they didn't have change for a £20 note! Don't mess with a woman in labour … I was not happy! I remember leaning against a tree when a contraction hit and not feeling that I could walk to the next shop.

My best friend came to visit me (and brought me paracetamol!) and I did my nails! The contractions were on and off all evening – they eventually got stronger later in the evening. I was coping well, but found I needed to be active. I likened the contractions to surfing – if you were ready for the wave and you caught it just right, you could just glide along on the top of it. But if you misjudged it, you would come crashing down and it hurt a lot.

Around midnight, something changed. I had some bleeding (which we later decided was just the rest of my show), the baby moved and the pain completely changed. I remember describing it as feeling like my back exploded. From then on, I had a constant pain in my back and at times couldn't even feel the contractions over the back pain. I later found out this was because the baby was 'back to back', with his spine rubbing against mine. It was agony. Once I saw the bleeding, combined with the constant pain, I panicked and we called the midwife. She came out and said I was around 4cm so I could go to the hospital. I said I'd had enough and wanted an epidural even before we left the house!

We got to the hospital, and my midwife filled an inflatable birthing pool and encouraged me to get in. I did and it was like a nice warm bath, and it was comfortable to lean against the side, but it did absolutely nothing to help my pain. I tried gas and air, but it just made me feel sick. At this point, I had really had enough and was just miserable verging on distressed. The labour completely slowed down, although I still had the constant back pain and couldn't get comfortable. I was exhausted. I felt at this point that they weren't ever going to let me have an epidural and that it was a conspiracy against me!

Eventually, around 6am, I got my epidural and that changed everything. She had to do it twice, but it then worked straight away. I went from being in complete agony to no pain at all. I suddenly felt back in control, which was a brilliant feeling. I did feel slightly like I had 'failed' the midwives by having an epidural, but to me this was pretty irrelevant as I was just so happy not to be in so much pain.

By this point, I was only 5cm dilated and they decided to put me on a drip to induce me and push the labour along. After this was in place, I was able to rest and even fell asleep. They woke me around midday, asking if I was ready to push. I felt rested, happy and in control. I had a small strip along the top of my belly where I could feel a contraction – this was really helpful as it gave me something to push against. I pushed for two hours. Around 2pm, they started to get concerned about the baby's heart rate. Although I was pushing the baby out, they recommended getting him out quicker using a ventouse. At that point the consultant and a few more people came into the room. They used the ventouse and very quickly the baby was out and they immediately laid him on me.

Throughout my pregnancy I had panicked about how I would feel about my baby (what if I don't like or love them?!), but for me that moment was incredible. I looked at him and remember thinking 'Oh, it's you! You're not at all scary!!!' I fell in love with him instantly and straight away said I'd have done it all again for him.

Anya's birth story

I had a pretty rotten time of it for my first birth. Second time round, I had to decide between a VBAC (vaginal birth after caesarean) or an elective caesarean.

One of the most powerful things that I was told by my midwife was, 'Whatever your decision, you must own it and go towards it with all your heart. Don't allow yourself or anyone else to question it.' That really helped me, and after discussions with the consultant I was booked in for a caesarean.

I went in at 38 weeks to meet with the consultant to ask if I could push my caesarean date back, to give my body a chance to go into labour naturally if that's what this baby wanted. The consultant patiently listened to me while she took my blood pressure. Then she responded, 'Well, I would certainly not suggest putting the date back. Your blood pressure is sky high and there's protein in your urine [signs of pre-eclampsia], so there might even be a case for having your baby today.' That was a bit of a shock (I didn't even have my hospital bag packed), but from that point on I felt a very calming sense that this was the way I was supposed to have my baby – there was no fighting it.

A week of blood pressure clinics followed, and I was measured for my attractive compression tights and given the pre-op meds. I closed my eyes on the last night when I had only one child. I slept fitfully, but excitedly. Next morning, my midwife texted at 8am saying 'Right, let's meet this baby!'

I was prepped for surgery at 9am. I had to don an attractive backless blue gown, and have all the pre-op checks with the anaesthetist team. It turned out there were staffing issues and a few electives had been pushed from the day before, so rather than being first, I was to wait indefinitely. I remember savouring the last few hours of being able to rub my tummy and feel my baby move around inside me, the last few moments where it was just me and him.

Finally, at 3pm, it was me. In my birth plan I had requested a 'natural caesarean', where the stages of natural birth are emulated as much as possible, with baby coming out gradually, head first, 'squeezed' by gentle pressure from the surrounding organs and tissue as if through the birth canal, which may help with draining the fluid in the lungs, which can be a problem with caesarean births. I imagined it being gentle and serene, to compensate for my loss of a natural birth.

In reality, I have a weak constitution when it comes to giving birth, and being sick is my modus operandi. It happened during my first labour, and this time all through the operation I was trying not to vom. I don't think I could've really cared less whether baby was being coaxed out gently or pulled out by his feet, I was just trying to keep on top of my waves of horrendous nausea. Twenty minutes later, the surgical team are still rummaging around inside me, which was really quite uncomfortable. It may not be a natural birth, but you can feel the sensations of tugging and pushing in your insides. Finally there is a hearty, angry scream and he's here!

I wanted to have skin-to-skin immediately, and my midwife placed Freddie in all his purple grimacing long-fingernailed glory onto my chest. In the recovery room, Freddie latched on perfectly – it helped that I was familiar with the logistics of feeding lying down as he was my second, but a caring midwife and skin-to-skin helped this to happen with no fuss, no crying.

It takes a good few hours for the anaesthetic to wear off, and in that time you have no feeling at all in your lower body. So, into the evening I was in the slightly ungainly position of a beached whale not being able to move at all, but I had my baby, and I felt so content. Even taking into account that I was being very sick for a very long time afterwards – lying down unable to move but regularly being sick into an NHS hospital bucket by your head, while your newborn is asleep at your boob, is pretty tricky. At 3am the nurse gave me an anti-nausea injection as it just wasn't abating. But I genuinely remember it as being a peaceful happy night on the postnatal ward. I felt very lucky that everything was okay, that my baby was okay.

11 Hey, baby!

The first few weeks with your newborn

SETTLING IN

It's a really good idea to read this section before you have your baby, for two reasons: first, it's good to be prepared for your headlong plummet into child rearing; and second, you won't have time to read anything once he's arrived!

> 'I would not recommend having family or overseas visitors within the first two weeks of having a new baby. Retrospectively, I think you need time to just stare and smell and glory in the wonder of your baby without having to get dressed.'
>
> Nicki

Assuming you had an uncomplicated vaginal delivery, you'll probably be dispatched from the maternity unit within about 12 hours of the birth. Some women just can't wait to get away; others rather enjoy the chance to lie in bed and be tended to for a while.

Once you're all installed at home, you may well find that anxiety strikes. It can feel weird, too – the fact that all of a sudden there's another person in the house, relying solely on you and your partner to love it, care for it and make sure it doesn't get damaged. Allow yourself plenty of time to adjust to all of this. It's a steep learning curve, and one you need to take at a steady pace.

If you're in any doubt about something, remember you don't have to tackle it alone: put in a call to your midwife or health visitor. If you can't get hold of someone quickly and you feel you need to, you can always call 111. It's a good idea to put all the important telephone numbers somewhere prominent, so you're not scrabbling around in a panic if you need them.

'I found the fourth trimester a really helpful concept – i.e. be kind to yourself and keep expectations really low initially. Baby has been inside you for nine months so it's a shock to both of you and cuddling baby all the time is absolutely okay. The first three months are just all about getting to know your baby, recovering and finding a new rhythm in life. Baby reaching three months was an important marker for me towards finding a new normal.'

Julie

FEEDING YOUR BABY

Getting enough nourishment into your new housemate is going to be one of your primary preoccupations over the coming weeks and months. On pages 184 and 187 I've covered the pros and cons of breastfeeding and bottle feeding. I want to reiterate now that how you feed your baby is your choice. There should be no stigma attached to either way.

Breastfeeding: the truth

I have breastfed my second baby in the following situations: in a sling while running after my three-year-old in a playground; on a bus; on the toilet; answering the door to the postman; while teaching a Pilates class. He's now 10 months old and I'm still breastfeeding – not right now … although, yes, come to think of it, I have also breastfed him while working on a computer ... Breastfeeding can be a seamless part of your life with your baby, and can offer you an immensely special feeling of intimacy, not to mention triumph that you alone are successfully feeding your baby and producing magic milk. Breastfeeding my second baby has been a journey of positive joy and simplicity. If you'd asked me what I thought about breastfeeding after my first baby, however, I would have given you a very different answer, as it was so, so hard and didn't really work – it was an emotionally and physically turbulent and difficult experience.

The simple truth is that breastfeeding is the most simple and natural thing in the world, and *when it works* it's the easiest, healthiest, not to mention most convenient way of feeding your baby (it's right there on tap, it's free, no bottles or faffing with sterilising equipment). But when it doesn't work, for whatever reason, it's very, very hard, particularly if you had had your heart set on breastfeeding, and you can feel like a failure as a mother if it's not going well. If you want to bottle feed and skip boob-feeding altogether, that's absolutely your choice and you should go ahead happily. If so, just skip the next few pages. If you do want to give breastfeeding a go, it's best to be prepared for the struggles that might lie in front of you, in order to be able to cope with them and get through them, nipples and sanity intact.

It might be that we simply aren't prepared for what breastfeeding involves, and assume that because it's natural we'll just know how to do it and it'll work from the off without any element of effort and practice – maybe that's why the early challenges prove too much for so many. Difficulty latching on, severely sore or infected nipples, poor milk supplies, or a disinterested or even distressed baby are all common problems, affecting even the steeliest resolve to feed your baby yourself. Statistics show that three-quarters of UK mums breastfeed initially, but less than a quarter are still giving their baby nothing but breast milk by six weeks, and, by six months, the optimum timeframe recommended by the Department of Health for breastfeeding, three-quarters have given up on it completely.

Some other books (and many health professionals) gloss over this bit, but I'm going to be upfront about it: when you're trying to get breastfeeding established, it can really, *really*, hurt. In a nutshell, be prepared for the first six weeks of breastfeeding to potentially be a challenge while you get to grips with it, and for the pain to be something that you just have to get through. If you can see past that, then you'll be able to envisage a long relationship feeding your baby. With my first I have to confess that there were times I actually dreaded putting him on the boob as it felt like someone was stabbing me with a knife – it felt worse than any pain of labour. They say that if it hurts, you're doing it wrong – but actually, it can really hurt if you're doing it right, too (initially, at least). And that's before you develop weals or cracks across the tender skin of your nipples, or worse – an infection – and you then have to put your infected or cracked nipple into the mouth of a hungry baby who will suck on it with no mercy. There are nipple shields easily available that can reduce the pain somewhat – I personally didn't get on with how they work, but I know others who have had a very successful experience with nipple shields to protect their assets and to not give up on breastfeeding.

'I wish I'd known more about skin-to-skin and breastfeeding. The NCT breastfeeding class was rubbish, and my son didn't latch and ended up not feeding, developing breathing problems and having 10 days in neonatal.'

Bella

The other thing that you're not always warned about with breastfeeding is the sheer amount of time you're likely to spend doing it at first. Very young babies don't half do a lot of demanding as their tummies are very tiny, so you can end up feeding every hour, for half an hour. Which is a lot, and your nips take the flak. Even with my second, who was a happy and effective feeder, the pain only began to subside fully after about two weeks. We spent a long time glued to the sofa feeding, with me watching TV in those early days – so always make sure you have the remote or a magazine, a tall glass of water, a cup of tea and a biscuit within reach when you settle down for a session. Feeding so often, and for so long in the early weeks, can make it seem as though you're spending nine and a half out of every 10 hours in a day pinned to the sofa. Eating cake. Breastfeeding entitles you to a lot of cake in those early weeks – but you deserve it, mama, and breastfeeding genuinely requires extra fuel! So if you're happy to, embrace it. It is a very small period of your life, in the grand scheme of things. Although it can feel like an eternity when you're in it.

The truth is that, once you've got it sussed, breastfeeding becomes a doddle: free, easy, lovely. I look back on the early weeks with my first, and I genuinely only linger on the memories of contentment with a snugly, smushy newborn at my breast, me gazing at him adoringly. I never find myself shuddering at the pain that I felt while getting the feeding established.

Usually, when it's going well, breastfeeding can be painful for a couple of weeks. If the pain doesn't settle down after those first two weeks, make sure you see someone soon, for your nerves as well as your nipples. Breastfeeding can take its toll on your emotional well-being if it's not going well and you persevere due to pressure on yourself or pressure from those around you. Be kind to yourself. Most early breastfeeding problems *can* be overcome if you're committed, and if you have the right support. So if you're struggling but determined, ask your midwife or health visitor to help. And if they don't have the time or inclination to help, make contact with a breastfeeding counsellor or lactation consultant – there'll be one in your area, or, at the very least, on the other end of the phone. There are lots of organisations dedicated to helping with breastfeeding, and they're listed at the back of the book.

‘Breastfeeding is natural but does not necessarily come naturally, and someone to help show the way to do it is so important. The flood of hormones moving through my body when I breastfed was also strange – I could actually feel them course through my body and feel my uterus cramp as it shrank back down.’

Ele

The importance of skin-to-skin

There are now a multitude of studies that show that mothers and babies should be together, skin-to-skin (baby naked, not wrapped in a blanket), immediately after birth. Baby is happier, her temperature is regulated, heart and breathing rates are more stable, and blood sugar is elevated. With skin-to-skin contact, baby starts to 'root' and search for the breast to show that she's hungry. It helps bubs breathe more naturally and stay warm in those hours immediately after birth when they're in the scary outside world for the first time.

From the point of view of breastfeeding, babies who have skin-to-skin with mum immediately after birth for at least an hour are more likely to latch on without any help, and, importantly, they are more likely to latch on properly. When baby latches on well, you're much less likely to be in a lot of pain. In the first few days, you'll be producing the first milk, colostrum, but until your milk comes in fully (hello rock-hard boobs), baby needs a good latch as she has to work quite hard to get it. When your milk properly 'comes in', baby can latch badly and potentially still get enough milk, although feedings may be long or frequent (or both), they'll be very painful, and you're more likely to develop problems such as blocked ducts and mastitis. Skin-to-skin early on helps to keep both of you calm, and there's more chance of baby instinctively knowing how to latch if you're both calm. And, let's face it, it's just pretty lovely having a smushy newborn lying on your naked skin so you can feel each other's heartbeat.

Don't forget – dads can also do skin-to-skin as an important part of the bonding process for him ... although it doesn't help his milk come in, thankfully.

Tips for successful breastfeeding

- Make sure you're comfortable. A footstool and a large pillow under your arm (or better still, a V-shaped breastfeeding cushion) can be a huge help. Cushions, cushions, cushions.

- Offer your baby the boob whenever he seems to want it. Although this can be exhausting, it's the best way to get your supply going – and it's not forever. Within a month or two, feeds will become speedier and more widely spaced – honest.

- Make sure your baby gets as big a mouthful of breast as possible, so he needs a big gape. If he seems not to be able to gape wide enough, have him checked immediately for tongue tie (see page 248). If he's just sucking at the end of your nipple, he won't be getting the milk out – and you'll be in a lot of pain. My lactation consultant likened it to my poor baby trying to drain a swimming pool with a straw. That ain't going to be easy for anyone.

- Unlatch baby and start again if it's wrong, and don't allow it to continue if you're in real pain after the first 30 seconds of suckling. But don't just pull away while he's still sucking for dear life, or you'll be in agony. Pop your little finger in the corner of his mouth to break the suction.

- Let your baby drain the whole breast before offering the other – and start the next feed with the last breast offered. (You'll know when it's empty because it will be soft and deflated.) Attach a safety pin or ribbon to your bra strap, and it will help you remember which breast you need to whop out first next time.

- Have lots of breast pads to hand. You won't believe how much milk can leak out.

- A natural remedy that really *does* ease sore and engorged boobs is cabbage leaves – although no-one is sure quite why – preferably chilled first in the fridge.

- It's best not to introduce a bottle or dummy while you're getting breastfeeding established, in case your baby becomes confused.

- If you're shy, you don't have to breastfeed in front of all and sundry. Find a quiet corner or ask for some privacy. A carefully draped muslin will help spare your blushes.

- Keep yourself well fed and watered while you're breastfeeding. Breastfeeding mums need about 400 calories more a day than when they were pregnant – so now you really do have an excuse to eat more cake. Continue to take 10mcg of vitamin D daily while breastfeeding, for the sake of your baby's bones and teeth.

- Don't smoke if you're breastfeeding, as the nicotine and other dangerous chemicals in tobacco smoke can be passed on to your baby.

- In theory, you should stick to the same sort of alcohol limits you did in pregnancy (although, if you can master the art of expressing, you can always freeze supplies of your breast milk for nights when you fancy a drink or three).

‘One of my friends who had three children, when I was pregnant for the first time, told me the best investment for her was a nice nursing bra as you pretty much wear them non-stop. This was one of my best bits of advice – they were the most expensive bras that I have ever bought but were super-comfortable and nice looking so I didn't just feel like a milk machine.’

Julia

Possible breastfeeding issues

As mentioned before, breastfeeding can bring with it many hurdles to overcome – here are a few common issues and what you can do about them. For more help, ask your midwife or attend a local breastfeeding clinic if you can.

Low milk supply

There is nothing more agonising than the feeling that, despite having the desire to, your body didn't get the memo and isn't producing enough milk. This is actually a 'thing' and can present itself in various scenarios. If you've had an exhausting birth experience or had a C-section, your body may have gone into slight shock, and this delays your milk coming in. Your baby may have an ineffective suck, or simply not the right technique, which means your breast isn't being drained fully and therefore the right signals aren't being sent to your body to produce more. This all happened to me first time round and it was a fairly demoralising and painful time. I wish I had asked for help sooner, so don't make the same mistake that I did.

What can you do? Well, there are things you can do but don't beat yourself up to the point of losing your rag. If you had your heart set on breastfeeding, please remember it's not the end of the world to give your baby a bottle of formula, no matter what your mother-in-law might imply. The main thing is that baby is fed. Beyond that, using a breast pump on top of feeding is a good way of stimulating your supply … as well as having your baby's latch checked by a specialist and simply putting your baby on the breast a lot. You end up feeling like a dairy cow, as most of your waking day (and night) is spent trying to produce milk, which is tiring, mentally and physically. So you need to drink loads of water and eat a lot of cake. Other things to try include taking a supplement of fenugreek, which is said to stimulate supply, and makes you smell a bit like a curry house. Check with your midwife or a lactation consultant for other tips. A good mantra for this 'dairy cow' time of life is: this too shall pass …

Tongue tie

It sounds like a method of medieval torture. In actual fact it's a surprisingly common issue. If your baby is struggling to feed, crying a lot and coming on and off the boob constantly during feeds, or if feeding is particularly agonisingly painful for you and feeding seems to be constant beyond the first couple of weeks, please immediately ask someone – your midwife, health visitor or a lactation specialist – to check for tongue tie. Tongue tie is a condition where the baby's tongue is basically attached to the bottom of her mouth by a piece of skin. Bit of a design flaw. Your baby's tongue needs to be able to draw your nipple fully into the back of her mouth, and if she doesn't have a wide enough gape in order to do this, then no amount of hours at the boob will ever get enough milk and it's a literal and figurative pain for both of you. It's very easy to spot and rectify – apparently, midwives in the olden days used to flick it with a sharp fingernail straight after birth. It's a slightly more regulated procedure now but make sure you get it seen to, as it really can make the difference between success and failure when it comes to breastfeeding.

Mastitis or blocked milk ducts

Mastitis is a really painful condition caused by inflamed breast tissue. It can be the result of a number of possible issues, such as your baby latching badly, not sucking effectively, or missing feeds. Symptoms are similar to flu: fever, shakes and you can feel really pretty crap. A visit to the doctor is a must if you suspect mastitis, as you'll need antibiotics. You can still feed while you're taking the antibiotics, and, perversely, continuing to feed might also help you get better as it will relieve the build-up of milk. But it is really painful and will be something that truly tests your breastfeeding resolve.

Cracked nipples

Oh, the pain. It's not fun, I'm not going to lie. Nipple cream does help, though, and can prevent it happening in the first place. Lansinoh is the brand you'll hear a lot about but basically any will do the job. Slather it on constantly – before and after feeds, overnight, in between feeds, after the shower, in the shower ... Keeping it in the fridge is a good tip for painful nips. It really is a godsend. Make sure you have some in every room. If you can, try to let your nipples have some air to heal as well in those first intense couple of weeks. This does require the ability to wander around with your boobs out, so you may not want to do it while Auntie Vera is visiting, but allow yourself the luxury of letting your boobs be free as much as possible in those early days and that will speed up your nipples' resilience.

Hitting the bottle

If you decided to bottle feed, or if breastfeeding doesn't take off for some reason and you've decided to go with bottles and formula, or expressed breastmilk, I repeat: don't beat yourself up about it, and ignore any disapproving health professionals or mothers-in-law. The formula for happy feeding, if you'll excuse the pun, is happy mummy = happy baby, happy baby = happy mummy. If breastfeeding isn't working for you and is tipping you into a downward slide, switch to the bottle! If boob wasn't ever on the agenda for you, don't feel guilty. The bottom line is that your baby is fed and growing nicely plumper by the day. That is what counts, ladies, no matter what breastfeeding tyrants might suggest.

As many a mum of a bouncing, bottle-fed baby will tell you, formula's a perfectly good alternative to breast milk, as long as you stick to the rules on hygiene and preparation. And it, too, has its advantages: it doesn't hurt; you can ask someone else to feed your baby for you (a big bonus in the middle of the night); you know exactly how much he's getting; and you won't ever have to get your boobs out in front of your father-in-law.

A bit of both

Remember that you can always 'combine feed': some bottle, some breast. Introducing a bottle tends to be easier the earlier you do it – hardly surprisingly, perhaps, as once a baby's accustomed to drinking sweet, warm breast milk from a nice, soft boob, a rubber teat and fake-tasting formula probably don't have the same appeal, so you might have to be persistent when it comes to introducing one. Once you've done so, though, you should find your baby will happily take from both – you can decide for yourself which feeds you want to be bottle and which breast, but you'll need to stick to the same method at the same times of the day, because of the supply-and-demand nature of the way the boobs work. One word of warning about mixed feeding, though: your boobs will quickly adjust to any new routine and a decreased demand. So if you start it, you'll fairly soon get to a point where you can't go back.

YOUR POST-BIRTH BODY

This is probably high on your list of worries – how on earth does your body return to normal after such an ordeal? Usually it will depend on what kind of birth you had. Some women get off lightly and find they recover within weeks, days even. For others, it may take months. To one degree or another, though, you're probably going to feel knackered and sore, albeit with the feeling of exhilaration that comes with having run a marathon. You did it! You brought a new person into the world! You're amazing. My motto to my postnatal Pilates mums is always: nine months in, nine months out. Give yourself proper time to recover from this pretty monumental event that your body has been through, and don't expect to ping back to normal immediately.

Once your little passenger is out, there are a few things you should expect to happen to your weary and wonderful body.

'My pelvic floor hurt for a long time afterwards, and my episiotomy cut too. Particularly as I was given painkillers in the hospital but not when I got home, so the pain was naturally worse at home too. But … nine months after Lara's birth, everything in my body is back to nearly how it was before.'

Maria

Bleeding

Known as lochia, the postnatal discharge of blood, mucus and tissue as the womb sheds its lining is experienced by every new mother. It varies from woman to woman, but you might find the amount somewhat alarming. 'I was really shocked by how long I bled for,' recalls *Modern Mum* Claire. 'I felt like it would never ever end. It became slightly depressing, like part of me was slowly but surely disappearing with each new day that brought more blood.'

Lochia is usually very heavy and bright red in colour for a few days but becomes lighter, changing to brown or pink, and will normally stop altogether within six weeks. If it returns to a bright red colour at any point, mention it to your midwife, as it could be a sign of infection, or that you're overdoing things. You'll need plenty of maternity pads to cope with the flow – tampons aren't a good idea because they could introduce infection into the vagina, and normal sanitary towels probably won't be up to the job. You should definitely tell your midwife if the bleeding doesn't slow after a few weeks, if it suddenly becomes extremely heavy or repeatedly clotted (some clots are normal), or if it starts to smell, as this could signal a problem.

Afterpains

Thought you'd felt your last contraction for a while during the birth? Erm, no, sorry – there are a few more to come. Your womb has to contract back to its normal size in the days after birth and this can be painful, particularly while breastfeeding, as it releases oxytocin, the hormone that triggers contractions. A painkiller such as paracetamol can help, as can a heat pack, or a hot water bottle.

Vagina and perineum

If you tore or had an episiotomy, you're going to be very sore indeed down below, and even if you didn't, it's likely to feel bruised and tender for a while – a fact you'll be painfully reminded of every time you sit down, or attempt to walk anywhere, probably in the manner of John Wayne.

If you had stitches, these may give you quite a bit of grief, with itchiness as well as pain compounding the misery. You can buy a range of products to help ease this discomfort, such as gel-filled packs which you chill and then pop in your pants, and anaesthetic sprays. Plain old painkillers and warm baths will usually offer relief, and some women reckon a drop or two of an appropriate essential oil such as lavender or tea tree can help, too. Arnica is widely believed to help relieve bruising and inflammation and boost the healing process, and some women swear by it. You can buy it in health food shops and most chemists, but make sure you read the label carefully before taking it.

Stitches can become infected, so your midwife will check them several times during her home visits to make sure they're healing without any problems. Try to keep the area clean – use a handheld shower to rinse a couple of times a day, especially after using the loo. Try using tissues rather than a towel, or even use a hairdryer (gives a whole new meaning to the term 'wash and blow dry' …). Change your pad regularly, making sure you wash your hands before and after. Tea tree and witch hazel are good for helping the wound to heal and for helping to prevent infection. Stitches will usually dissolve on their own after a week or two, but sometimes they may need to be taken out.

Soreness down below makes going to the loo after birth a major trial. Having a wee can sting like buggery – it helps to tinkle just before you get out of the bath, or pour warm water over your bits in mid-flow. Drink plenty of fluids, as this will reduce the concentration of your urine and make it sting less.

Doing your pelvic floor exercises will help healing, as it increases blood flow to the area, so do get cracking on these as soon as you can bear to. Turn back to page 120 to remind yourself how.

It's a grim thought, but if you're unlucky enough to experience a more extensive tear (known as a third- or fourth-degree tear), you could end up suffering from bowel problems. Pelvic floor exercises will be particularly important, and you can be referred to an obstetric physiotherapist for specialist help.

'I had a third-degree tear and I felt like I'd been ripped in two – the pain was off the scale and I couldn't sit down. I spent days in tears after the birth. I had no idea that it would be so debilitating.'

Hannah

Assuming everything's okay, you'll get the go-ahead from your doctor to have sex again six weeks after birth (although it's all right to try before that, if you're in good shape below, your lochia flow has ceased – and you can find the energy). In reality, many women don't feel up to it, for psychological as well as physical reasons, for several months or more.

You might also worry about the way your vagina looks and feels after childbirth, perhaps fearing you've been left with something of a 'wizard's sleeve' down there. It's true that elasticity can be reduced, and that raised scar tissue may have changed its appearance, which can make things feel and look a little different down there. But most couples find these to be minor details. If you're really worried that things aren't right after a period of time, definitely have a chat to your GP.

Bowels and bum

Trying to do a poo in the days after birth can become a trauma of rather large proportions, not helped by the fact that the bowels can become sluggish after birth anyway, because the muscles and nerves down there have come in for such a bashing. 'Two days post-birth I finally had a poo,' recounts *Modern Mum* Hannah. 'It was horrendous, like giving birth all over again.'

In fact, it's highly unlikely you'll rip open your stitches, but it might feel as if you're going to. Holding a maternity pad or a clean wedge of tissues over the stitches should give you the psychological reassurance you need to go for it. Constipation will make things worse (and this can lead to a bit of a vicious circle), so keep up your fibre intake and drink plenty of water. If necessary, ask your midwife to recommend a gentle laxative treatment. And bear in mind that, although many women dread the first bowel movement, in reality it probably won't be as bad as you fear.

Piles are common after birth, caused by the pressure of the delivery on your anus, and can make for yet more painful, itchy misery. You can buy over-the-counter treatments that offer some relief, and if they're really bad your midwife will be able to get a suppository prescribed for you. But they should go away on their own after a while.

⁶I think you just need to adjust expectations – your body has done something extraordinary in creating a baby and it will never go back to exactly what it was, but it doesn't need to either. In terms of fitness, I would say take it easy. I felt like my insides were going to drop to the floor when I went for my first run so I would recommend focusing

intently on pelvic floor exercises and take little steps initially to get you to your long-term goal.'

Nicki

Boobs

A couple of days after birth, your milk 'comes in', and you will wake up to discover that you have two unbearably tender breasts that are suddenly the size and texture of granite boulders. It's caused by a big hormonal surge and won't last longer than a couple of days.

If you're breastfeeding, the best way to relieve the pain and pressure this causes is to feed your baby – although you may find you have to gently express a little at first (try massaging them while you're in the bath) so they're not too full for him to get his mouth round. And yes, it's an irony: the biggest boobs you've ever had and the only person reaping the benefits is your baby. That's life.

You might also feel that your milk coming in – which happens regardless of whether you want to breastfeed or not – is accompanied by feelings of the flu with a slight fever and shakes. Pay attention to these symptoms because, although normal, they can also be signs of mastitis, particularly if any red patches appear on your breast. Mastitis is a condition that causes the breast tissue to inflame painfully and may need treatment – if so, it needs to be dealt with through a course of antibiotics, so do see your midwife or GP if you start to feel really unwell.

'I would have loved to know before that it's common to have shakes in the days after birth. In the middle of the night I started to shake uncontrollably, my teeth chattering in a way I really couldn't stop. When I finally managed to shout loud enough for my boyfriend to hear I was beside myself. We called the hospital and they asked my boyfriend to check a few things, which were all fine. It wasn't an infection, but rigors, which can apparently happen when milk comes in, but they're not commonly talked about.'

Manna

If you're not breastfeeding, there'll be a painful few days while the milk subsides (and it should have dried up completely within a few weeks). You'll need a snug-fitting bra, and possibly some paracetamol, to ease your way through this period.

Belly

Your tummy will still be big for a while, only it won't be firm and round anymore – it'll be as wobbly as blancmange and probably you'll still have a bump that looks around five months pregnant in the immediate aftermath of the birth. Don't, whatever you do, worry about this during the first few months – there'll be time enough in the future to get back into your old jeans – and it's certainly not a good idea to start working out during the first six weeks. If you've had a caesarean, you'll need to be patient for longer, and you may have quite an alarming 'overhang' above the scar site. This will go down in time, so be kind to yourself.

However, if you want to make a tentative start on getting some strength back in your abdomen, you can, by gently pulling in your tummy and holding it for a few seconds before releasing, whenever you get the chance. Remember to have your tummy checked for diastasis recti – this is where the abdominal muscles split to accommodate your growing baby. It's very common, and, in my experience teaching postnatal Pilates, many women have it postnatally without realising it – sadly, it's not an automatic part of the GP's six-week check for some crazy reason. Diastasis recti happens during most pregnancies. And it's more common than not to still have a small gap immediately postnatally. Usually, the tummy muscles repair within the first couple of months without you doing anything specific. But, if you've had a big baby, or depending on the strength of your abdominal muscles pre-pregnancy, this isn't always the case and you're left with a gap after baby has left its former residence. Get it checked: ask your GP, midwife or a trained exercise professional. If undetected, an abdominal gap can get worse and, in rare cases, only surgery will help knit the muscles back together. A qualified Pilates instructor can help you mend your abdominals safely.

'When my son was a year old I still looked five months pregnant. I started Pilates and started learning about diastasis recti, muscle separation in the abdomen, which many people have during pregnancy, but usually the muscles close themselves and you're none the wiser. Mine, though, had been so ripped apart by big babies, they couldn't recover without surgery.'

Hannah

As for stretch marks, if you have them, they'll fade eventually – although they won't go altogether. There are lots of lotions and potions on the market at varying prices that claim to help, but since none are proven to have dramatic effects, you may as well stick to inexpensive cocoa butter or vitamin E-based brands if you're keen to give one a go. Meanwhile, lots of women swear by fake tan as a means of covering up the worst of their 'baby battle scars' or 'tiger stripes'.

Serious post-birth symptoms

There are some post-pregnancy symptoms that could signal a serious complication or infection, so don't hesitate to give your midwife or GP a shout if your bleeding becomes very severe; if you feel faint, dizzy or feverish; if there's any swelling, tenderness or pain in your legs; if you can't shake a severe headache, particularly if it comes with vomiting or blurred vision; if you have a persistent pain in the tummy or down below; or if you're having a lot of pain when weeing.

Weak or leaky bladders

Don't be surprised if you're finding it hard to keep urine in – weak and leaky bladders are another common and delightful consequence of giving birth. Doing your pelvic floor exercises will help (everyone should do them after birth, anyway, to avoid problems in the future). And you're not excused just because you had a C-section – pregnancy in itself puts a strain on your pelvic floor, so you could still be at risk. If the problem's really bad, or persists beyond a few weeks, tell your doctor. They may refer you to a specialist for treatment.

RECOVERY AFTER A CAESAREAN SECTION

A caesarean section is major abdominal surgery, and so it will take longer to recover from than a straightforward vaginal birth. How long that will be varies. You should have got over the worst after six weeks, but some women say they still don't feel right for up to a year afterwards. Recovery from an emergency C-section is likely to take longer than if you had an elective. I have had two caesareans: one was an emergency after having laboured for three days, and the second was an elective. My recoveries could not have been more different. Worlds apart: from awful (first) to brilliant (second). So, every birth and every caesarean is different.

‘If you've had a C-section, wear *big pants*, and don't overdo it. I was like a beetle on its back for days as none of my muscles were working and it hurt everywhere!’

Bella

- You'll usually have to stay in hospital for three to four days, on average, and you'll need some heavy-duty painkilling medication. You'll be given a good supply of pain relief medication to take home with you, too, and probably some blood-thinning injections to administer yourself over the next few days to limit the chance of blood clots, which is a bit alarming. There's nothing like having to jab your own postnatal wobbly belly with a massive needle to make you feel like insult is being added to injury.

- You'll probably find even simple activities, such as sitting up or walking, hard work, and will need lots of help and support (if you're on your own, you may need a good friend or relative to come and stay with you for a while).

- There's no reason why you can't cuddle and breastfeed your baby – I was feeding my second within an hour of giving birth to him – although you may need a little help in working out how to do so comfortably.

- As it will really hurt to cough, sneeze or laugh, ask for someone at hospital to show you how to do so without it causing trouble for your incision site. You can now buy caesarean belts to help cushion and protect the area post-birth.

- It's common to suffer from painful trapped wind after a caesarean, as your digestive system may have been affected by the surgery – I would liken this pain almost to an early contraction in terms of intensity. It really hurts, so breathing through it works, just as it does for contractions. Peppermint tea is widely recommended as a means of relief.

- Don't panic if your incision site looks very obvious or vivid at this point – it will shrink and fade to a fine, pale line with time. You may suffer from some itchiness around the area and it's a good idea to keep it clean and dry. The stitches will either dissolve or need removing at a later stage.

- Dress in very loose comfortable clothing for a while. In particular, you're going to need some very roomy pants.

- You'll be warned not to drive for at least a couple of weeks after having a C-section: make sure you are able to twist comfortably enough to do up your seat belt and reverse the car. These are the movements that you may struggle with until your abdominals have healed sufficiently (your insurance company may insist on six weeks – check the small print). And avoid lifting anything heavy for several months.

- Women who've had an unplanned, emergency C-section may find it hard to deal with emotionally. They might be disappointed because they didn't get the natural birth they planned, or even feel that they've 'failed' to have a 'proper' birth. Or they may be traumatised by whatever happened during labour to trigger the need for a caesarean, particularly if it was anything to do with fetal distress. When things take a turn for the worse to whatever degree, there is a real feeling of lack of control and it can be very upsetting. One way to deal with this is to go over what happened during the birth, and talk about it a lot, with someone who is sympathetic (see below).

YOUR POSTNATAL CARE

In most areas you'll remain under the care of a community midwife for around 10 days, and she should arrange to drop in on you several times during this period to make sure both you and your baby are doing okay. After this time, your health visitor – a qualified nurse or midwife who works in the community with families – will take over. Exactly how many visits you get will depend on policy, how pressed they are, and how much you need them.

Your baby should get a full medical once-over within three days of his birth – this could either be when you're still in hospital or once you get home, usually by a visiting GP. His length and weight measurements will be taken, and checks made on his eyes, heart, hips and (boys only, naturally) testes. A week or so after the birth, your midwife will want to do a heel prick test on your newborn. It's a routine screening process which involves taking a small sample of blood from your baby's heel, which is then sent away to check for a number of rare but serious conditions.

And these days, all babies get a routine hearing test soon after birth, too – it's a very quick, simple test that involves a small earpiece being put in your baby's ear for a few moments.

'In the weeks and months after birth I felt very overwhelmed – it was also lonely. I would not have got through so well without my new NCT pals – we formed a really supportive group. I always knew that, even when I was up eight times a night, I could text someone and they would be there too. Step away from Google – Google is not your friend at 3am. Trying to have confidence in your own gut feeling is something to treasure – you are probably right.'

Becca

The alien has landed

Wondering if you have in fact given birth to an alien? Or which one of you he inherited that strange-shaped head from? Fear not. Newborn babies are weird little beings, with many mysterious features. Here are some random facts about them that may surprise you.

- Their first poos (meconium) are dark and sticky. The dark sticky stuff will soon give way to something yellow or green and runny (in breastfed babies) but paler and firmer (and generally smellier) if formula-fed.

- Their skin is very often flaky, blotchy, rashy or spotty. (Check with your health visitor if you're worried, but in most cases it will be harmless and normal.)

- They may be very hairy. This is the remains of lanugo, the covering that protected them in the womb, and will drop out soon.

- They may also still have vernix on them, and so be a bit greasy. Don't bother trying to wash it off – it'll help protect against dry skin.

- Their heads may be a weird shape, squished by the journey down the birth canal (and especially if vacuum extraction or forceps were used to ease them out). The soft spot on the top, where the skull bones have yet to fuse, is called the fontanelle. It's likely to be a year or more before it closes up. In the meantime, you don't have to be neurotic about damaging it – there's a tough layer of membrane underneath the skin which you'd really have to go some to penetrate.

- Their eyes may squint. This is because the muscles around them have yet to develop.

- The remains of the umbilical cord stay attached to their bellies for a few weeks after birth, after which it shrivels and drops off, leaving you with a delightful souvenir of their early weeks. In the meantime, keep a careful eye on it and let your midwife or health visitor know if it looks sore, as it can sometimes become infected.

- Their genitals and nipples may be swollen, due to hormones passed on by you. If you have a little girl, she may have a little blood in her nappy for the same reason.

- They are very likely to chuck up a large amount of milk when you feed them. This is known as possetting. It's normal, but check with your health visitor if it seems truly copious, is projectile or a strange colour, or if they seem to be in pain.

- They may sleep for hours and hours on end during the day in the first few weeks. Make the most of the time to catch up on some rest yourself!

Your midwife will want to make sure you're doing okay, too. When she comes, she'll examine your belly to make sure your womb is returning to normal, and check your stitches to see if they're healing and that there's no sign of infection. She'll look at your legs for signs of a blood clot (see page 37); check your temperature and blood pressure; and make sure your blood loss is normal. She'll also want to know that your bowel and bladder movements are okay. She may also ask you about contraception; although your immediate reaction may be to snort with laughter, it's worth bearing in mind, since it's technically possible to conceive just three weeks after giving birth – even if you *are* breastfeeding.

Both you and your baby will also be offered a more comprehensive check-up, usually with a GP or practice nurse, six to eight weeks after the birth.

BABY-CARE ESSENTIALS

This is, as you've hopefully gathered, a pregnancy book. But here's a very basic outline of baby-care essentials so you can read, prepare and digest this info before the baby comes. For more detailed information through the first year, try *First-Time Mum* (White Ladder, 2012).

Washing your baby

There's no reason why you can't put your baby in the big bath from the start, but as this can sometimes freak them out a little at first, you might be better off just to 'top and tail' them in the early weeks. You don't even need a baby bath for this: a clean washing-up bowl of cooled, boiled water will do just fine. Undress him, wrap him in a towel to keep warm, and then gently wipe his eyes, face, neck and around the ears (not inside), around the cord stump, hands and nappy area. Watch out in particular for dribbles of milk gathering in folds under the neck and armpits – some babies have been known to produce cheese under here! Dry him, creases too, by gently patting with a towel.

Changing your baby

Changing your baby's nappy straight away after she's done a poo, or whenever it's getting a bit soggy, will help prevent nappy rash. Clean and dry her bottom thoroughly (cotton wool and water's usually recommended, but alcohol-free baby wipes won't cause any harm), and apply a little barrier cream. It's important to keep a close eye on her bottom business: wet nappies are a good sign she's feeding well. Generally speaking, she should be producing six to eight wees over 24 hours. As for poo, the habits of breast-fed babies can be wildly erratic, and it's nothing to worry about if they go for several days without one. Formula-fed babies are more prone to constipation, so you should mention it to a health visitor or midwife if yours hasn't done a poo for more than a day. If you see any crystals in the nappy in the early days, and the nappies are not very wet, ask your midwife or health visitor for advice as these can be indications that your baby is dehydrated.

'I was lucky to have some people I really got on with in my NCT group and that we could be honest about the relentlessness of the early weeks. Most people were pretty honest about the fact their babies were erratic, didn't feed or sleep when they were supposed to, and often cried for no reason whatsoever.'

Julia

Holding your baby

It's normal to feel scared about this at first, since new babies are just so small, floppy and delicate. You'll soon work out how he most likes to be held, but, meanwhile, the most important thing to remember is to support his head, as babies have no strength in their neck muscles for the first few months. A friend visited when my second was four weeks old, and, obviously more used to and comfortable with older children, he proceeded to swing my little one in the air and do 'flying baby' – I had to remind him, quite forcefully, that he was only four weeks and couldn't actually hold his head up properly …!

Why won't he stop crying?

Some parents are flabbergasted by how much their new baby cries – between one and three hours a day of wailing is quite normal – and, very often, it's for no discernible reason. My first was a crier: oh man, he could cry, and cry, and cry – hence the haunted look in my eyes that lingers there still.

Though mystifying and distressing, it's not unusual to have a baby who cries excessively – up to a fifth of babies are believed to suffer from the tendency (although, frankly, it's the parents who come off worst). Excessive crying is usually called colic, which seems a very inadequate way of dismissing what can be a truly traumatising experience if your baby seriously does cry All. The. Bleedin'. Time. As my first did. No-one's really sure why exactly it happens, although there are plenty of theories – the most popular is that it's due to pain caused by an immature digestive system, although some say it's the baby freaking out as the reality of life outside the womb hits home. It's worth reminding yourself that it's never because your baby doesn't like you – it's hard, but try not to take it personally or think it's something you've 'done'. And my crier has turned into a perfectly content and smiley child, so it is a short-lived pain.

If your baby's crying relentlessly, it's important first to rule out any possible triggers by checking he's not hungry, tired, in need of changing, or poorly.

If it's none of those things, then all you can do is work your way through a list of potential solutions, which will usually include holding your baby close, cuddling, jiggling, rocking, swinging, shhhhing or singing. A walk in the pushchair or sling can work wonders, and the fresh air will do you good too. With some babies, a drive in the car is the only thing that can help. And many parents swear by a vibrating chair.

There are various commercial preparations, such as Infacol, that are said to help with colic, and we had some success with gripe water – these won't definitely stop the crying, but you may feel it's worth a shot. Some theorise that baby massage or cranial osteopathy – an alternative therapy that involves the application of light pressure, in an attempt to reduce tension within the body – is the answer. Baby massage is a wonderful way of allowing any trapped wind to be, er, expelled from the body, so either join a baby massage course, which in itself is a fun bonding thing to do with your newborn, or check out YouTube for baby massage demonstrations. The 'bicycle legs' manoeuvre got my baby farting, which definitely helped his comfort. Cranial osteopathy also helped my grouchy baby – it turned out he had a whole lot of tension and possibly residual pain from his birth experience. I was in labour for nearly three days and then he had to be whipped out by C-section as his heart rate had slowed. Thinking about it, it was probably just as stressful an experience for him as it was for me, so no wonder the poor thing was a cranky little soul for his first few months. Remember that the only way tiny babies can communicate their needs to you is crying. Trouble is, it's now your job to decipher what the hell they're trying to say.

Do check with your health visitor or GP if you have a problem with a relentlessly crying baby, as once in a while there'll be a medical reason for their distress. For me, excessive crying helped ultimately to flag up the fact that he wasn't feeding effectively and was essentially just very, very hungry. It led us to have him checked for tongue tie, go to a cranial osteopath, and switch to combined feeding after trying to exclusively breastfeed – and the combination of all of these three things meant that within a couple of weeks he was an utterly changed baby.

However, in most cases, infuriatingly, you'll probably be told to grin and bear it. This is a time for the 'this too shall pass' mantra. Please believe me when I say it's a short-term problem: it *will* stop, and your sanity *will* return. The good news about colic is that it almost always eases up by the time your baby is about three months old, which is not so long in retrospect (although it's true that it may as well be three years if you're in the thick of it). There are organisations you can call if it's getting too much for you, such as Crysis, which provides support for families with excessive criers, or sleepless and particularly demanding babies (details in the Useful Contacts section). It can be a very isolating experience, having a sleepless crier, especially if you look around and all other babies you see appear to be content and serene. So do reach out for help.

If in doubt, walk out

It's normal to have feelings of anger and desperation sometimes, if you have a baby who cries a lot. And I know only too well – I've been there. When you get to a point where you've reached the end of your tether, try to enlist help from someone else until you can feel calm again – or, if there's no-one around, put your baby in his cot and leave the room for a few moments and take some deep breaths. Make yourself a cup of tea, or pour a glass of wine. Phone a friend if need be. Your baby will come to no harm left crying for a short period. And when you need a break, you need a break.

Oh, the sleepless nights …

When they're not feeding, new babies usually sleep (let's face it, there's not much else to do, really, at that age). Unfortunately, this pattern of sleeping and feeding just carries on over 24 hours, so that day isn't really any different from night. You can fully expect to be woken four or more times by a new baby wanting sustenance, and probably a nappy change while you're at it. There's not a lot to be done about it but pander to the wee insomniac's needs. Things do settle down and night wakings will (usually) become less frequent over the coming months. And later still, from when your baby is around six months old, there are techniques that will help her sleep through the whole night if you can't take the broken nights any more. Until then, you'll just have to accept you're going to be a walking zombie for a while. Tip: bright red lipstick detracts from a tired eye. True story.

'Emotionally, when there were bad days, they were intense. On a bad day you think: this is it. This is my life, forever. I now have this baby stuck to me 24/7. Feeding every hour and not sleeping much. I look horrendous, have aged 10 years in 10 days, and there is no going back. I am unable to leave the house on time, none of my clothes fit me and I have no energy. And this is it; going forward it will ALWAYS be like it is now. And this is the error. As, of course, it will not be; it will change for the better.'

Beatriz

Safe sleeping

Cot death is rare, thankfully. But in the UK 300 babies a year still die suddenly and unexpectedly in their sleep. No-one knows why for certain, but there are a great many factors that increase the risk, and lots of measures you can take to reduce it. In a nutshell, though, here are the golden rules.

- Put your baby to sleep on his back, 'feet to foot', with his feet at the foot of the cot.

- Make up his bedding at the foot of the cot (so he can't wriggle down under his covers).

- Make sure he's not overdressed (a single vest and sleepsuit's fine), and the room isn't too hot (16°C to 20°C is ideal – you can get a room thermometer for a few quid from FSID (Foundation for the Study of Infant Deaths), but they're often given free with baby magazines or when you buy other equipment.

- Don't put too much bedding on – one blanket's usually enough, and no hats.

- Don't fall asleep with your baby on a sofa or chair, and think carefully before having your baby in bed with you. Most experts advise against co-sleeping in any circumstances, but if you really want to have your baby in bed with you, make sure you follow the guidelines given by UNICEF, which aim to minimise the risks: don't co-sleep if you or your partner (or both of you) smoke; if either of you has been drinking or taking any other mind-altering substance; if your baby is very small or was premature; or if you are 'unusually' tired. Don't ever put your baby under the covers or have a lot of pillows and bedding around. If in doubt, talk to your midwife or health visitor. You can buy 'safe' co-sleeper cots and baby nests that let you sleep safely with your baby in the bed next to you. Details are in the Useful Contacts section.

- Don't smoke near your baby – or anywhere in the house. Carbon monoxide is exhaled on the breath for several hours following each cigarette and it can linger on clothing, and there's a very strong link between smoking and cot death. If you haven't given up by now, you really should.

- Keep your baby's crib or cot in your room with you, for at least the first six months.

HOW YOU'LL FEEL

There's a general view that once you've had a baby, life is sweet. It certainly can be. But it's normal to feel a real mixed bag of emotions initially, with the lows as common as the highs. An attack of the 'baby blues' affects the vast majority of women during the early days or weeks after birth, and while these are often blamed on a surge of hormones, they're just as likely to be a simple reaction to an exhausting birth experience, lack of sleep or overwhelming change. Baby blues generally pass quickly and are best tackled with rest, cuddles and a good cry. But keep an eye on them: for up to one in five women they may give way to postnatal depression, a more serious condition that typically kicks in a month or two down the line, and can take a severe emotional toll. Having good perinatal mental health is really important for you and your baby; more and more maternity units now have a Perinatal Mental Health team, who should be able to offer, or signpost you to a wide range of psychological therapies, support groups and well-being sessions. At least one in 10 women get perinatal mental health problems, so don't be scared or slow to ask for help,

‘My tip: spend the first week alone with your partner and your new baby. Short visits are okay but definitely not overnight visits. I felt really, really sad for days but I couldn't really explain why, even to my partner. The sadness goes away again. I can't say that anything special helped. Apart from crying when you need to, and lots of rest.’

Maria

Also, far beyond the mild ups and downs of baby blues is birth trauma, which can occasionally affect women who are left seriously shaken by birth itself. This is considered by experts to be a form of post-traumatic stress disorder. If it is something that affects you, do confide in a sympathetic health professional, as it's really important that you get some help with it. Talking through your birth experience is reckoned to be a positive thing to do – your hospital may offer a service that allows you to go in and get any 'unresolved feelings' off your chest – this is often known as 'debriefing' or 'birth reflections'. Or, you may be able to get some counselling.

I can say from experience that, although you can and should hold onto the fact that your baby was born healthy and 'all was fine in the end', a traumatic birth experience does cut quite deeply and can have a negative effect on your first months of motherhood, and future pregnancies may even be affected by any emotional fallout that you end up suppressing. I didn't realise after my first, pretty awful, birth that you could request a debriefing to go through your maternity notes and labour experience with a consultant midwife, so I didn't do this until I became pregnant again. But it answered so many questions and made me feel differently about lots of things that I had otherwise been questioning and beating myself up about, I wish I had known and done it sooner. Talking about your experience, or in some other way offloading and sharing, is definitely a way of minimising the potential long-term negative effects of a traumatic birth.

> 'I have a vivid memory of what I can only describe as a post-traumatic moment when the reality of the childbirth experience came back to me and I was suddenly very upset and a bit panicky. It was a kind of delayed reaction.'
>
> Natalie

Bonding with your baby

It's not always love at first sight. Plenty of new mums look down at the baby they've just produced and feel pretty blank. As *Modern Mum* Maria recalls: 'I felt a bit lonely. Then I felt like I'd run a marathon; everything hurt. I also felt relieved, that everything went well. But for me the big feeling of over-flowing love for my child was missing at the beginning. For the first days in hospital I was happy that there were nurses on call, whenever needed. I felt a bit clueless.'

Give yourself time – you'll almost certainly be flooded with feelings of love for your baby at some point, soon. If not, then don't be afraid to talk to your midwife about it. It could be that you're suffering from postnatal depression and for that, you'll need some kind of help.

Taking it easy

The best piece of advice I can give you is to take it easy straight after you've had your baby. In Chinese medicine there is the ancient concept of 'doing the month' after you've had a baby. You stay in your home, attended to by your family, and you simply rest. For a whole month. We've largely lost that notion in the west and are more likely to be found zipping around the supermarket within days of having a baby. It makes sense to try to tap into the hugeness of the event that your body has been through, and give yourself time to recover, heal and bond with your new family. You've got a lot on your plate, what with the physical recovery from birth and the emotional adjustment to parenthood to make. Lean on your partner and/or anyone else who's around and is willing to give you support at this time. Let the housework go (although a little attention to basic hygiene is probably sensible) and eat ready meals and snacks if you need to.

‘What they say about just leaving the housework and relaxing with baby is SO TRUE, but no-one does it. You really won't remember dirty plates and laundry, but you will remember how you feel in those first precious weeks. I really regret that I didn't just sit gazing at my baby. I carried on as normal, tidying and busying myself in case visitors minded the mess. I will never again have a newborn and no other responsibilities so won't ever get to do it – so spend the whole day in your PJs, watch box sets, get REST and sleep when the baby does!’

Bella

Visitors will obviously be keen to come and you may well be happy to see them. But absolutely don't offer to cook or make tea for them (ask them to bring *you* food) and don't be afraid to politely but firmly impose a time limit on their stay. There's nothing worse than visitors lingering on your sofa for hours when you're desperately trying to establish breastfeeding. Obviously, if it's a good friend or a close relative who you enjoy having around and who's prepared to make themselves useful, then that's fine. On the other hand, if a mother-in-law is making your life miserable by staring at you every time you try to breastfeed, or offering unsolicited advice that you could, frankly, do without, you should probably ask them to leave – or give them an 'important' job to do in a different room.

When my second baby was four days old we inadvertently became hosts to a full family party when there were 10 people in our home, all sitting and taking turns to hold my sleeping newborn while I somehow ended up making tea for everyone. They all chatted and gossiped, didn't tell me I looked fantastic once (you will soon become aware that it's an unwritten rule that all visitors must tell you that you look amazing, even if you're in your pyjamas at 4pm, have skydiver hair and haven't worn make up for days, revealing the full extent of your sleeplessness), and then they all trotted off when the tea and (my) cake ran out, leaving me with a now fully awake and crying newborn. I don't advise this type of experience in the early weeks after your birth – it really is energy depleting at a time when you most need to keep your reserves up. Keep it low-key, rest, and only welcome visitors who are going to nurture and support you – and, most importantly, bring you unlimited supplies of tea and biscuits (or a lasagne to place in your freezer for some day in the not-too-distant future when your partner is back at work and you're in charge of the baby on your own for the first time, wondering how on earth it's supposed to all come together). It gets easier, I promise.

'The most important thing, though, I think is to stay connected, whether it be with an NCT group or just family and friends. Babies take up a lot of time and energy but they won't ever say thank you and you need other people to acknowledge that what you are doing is incredible, hard, tough and relentless, and that you are doing it brilliantly.'

Nicki

Above all, spend this time getting to know your baby and make the most of this undeniably special period in your baby's life. Before you know it, he's going to be a hulking great toddler, ripping your house apart at the seams and challenging your parenting skills with a whole new set of unfathomable behaviours. Enjoy your sweet serene newborn while he can't answer back. Remember: the intensity of these first few weeks does fade into a new normal, and there is a parental amnesia about the hard stuff that kicks in, to promote the extension of the human race. One day, you'll be watching your one-year-old walking around the living room with a washing basket on her head, laughing until your cheeks hurt. And the thought will enter your head, 'Wouldn't it be nice to have another …'

Useful contacts

Alcohol and smoking

Information and advice on alcohol consumption: www.drinkaware.co.uk

Online help to quit smoking: quitnow.smokefree.nhs.uk

Pregnancy stop-smoking helpline: 0300 123 1044

Birth

Aromatherapy: www.aromatherapycouncil.co.uk

Association for Improvements in the Maternity Services: www.aims.org.uk

Birth choice – where to have your baby: www.birthchoiceuk.com

British Acupuncture Council: www.acupuncture.org.uk; 020 8735 0400

Caesarean information and support on all aspects of caesareans: www.caesarean.org.uk

Caesarean procedure and mother's rights information: www.csections.org

Doula UK: www.doula.org.uk; 0871 433 3103

Home birth: www.homebirth.org.uk

Hypnobirthing: www.hypnobirthing.co.uk; www.natalhypnotherapy.co.uk; www.hypnobirthingandbeyond.com

Independent midwives: www.imuk.org.uk; 0300 111 0105

Induction information: www.nhs.uk/conditions/pregnancy-and-baby/pages/induction-labour.aspx

National Childbirth Trust (NCT): www.nct.org

Reflexology: www.aor.org.uk; 01823 351010

Breastfeeding

La Leche League helpline: 0845 120 2918

National Breastfeeding Helpline: 0300 100 0212

NCT breastfeeding helpline: 0300 330 0771

Childcare

National Day Nurseries Association: www.ndna.org.uk; 01484 40 70 70

Professional Association for Childcare and Early Years:

www.pacey.org.uk; 0300 003 0005

Employment

Department for Work and Pensions: www.gov.uk

GOV.UK – official government website: www.gov.uk

Shared parental leave: www.gov.uk/shared-parental-leave-and-pay/overview

Working Families: www.workingfamilies.org.uk; 0300 012 0312

Exercise

Guild of Pregnancy and Postnatal Exercise Instructors: www.postnatalexercise.co.uk

Food safety

British Dietetic Association: www.bda.uk.com

Food Standards Agency: www.food.gov.uk

Health in pregnancy, including diet and nutrition: www.tommys.org

Pregnancy information service: 0870 777 3060

General information and support

Baby Centre: www.babycentre.co.uk

Bounty parenting club: www.bounty.com

Co-sleeping – safe co-sleeping guidelines: www.nct.org.uk/parenting/co-sleeping-safely-your-baby

Cry-sis – offers support for families with excessively crying, sleepless and demanding babies: www.cry-sis.org.uk

Emma's Diary – baby and pregnancy advice: www.emmasdiary.co.uk

HSE (Health and Safety Executive): www.hse.gov.uk

Maternal Mental Health Alliance: maternalmentalhealthalliance.org.uk

Midwives Online: www.midwivesonline.com

Mumsnet – parenting network: www.mumsnet.com

National Childbirth Trust (NCT): www.nct.org

Netmums – parenting website: www.netmums.com

NHS Choices: www.nhs.uk

NICE (National Institute for Health and Care Excellence): www.nice.org.uk

Pregnancy and birth helpline: 0300 3300 772

Royal College of Obstetricians and Gynaecologists: www.rcog.org.uk

Losing a baby

Ectopic pregnancy: www.ectopic.org.uk; 020 7733 2653

Miscarriage: www.miscarriageassociation.org.uk; 01924 200 799

Medical conditions

Obstetric cholestasis: www.icpsupport.org

Pelvic girdle pain: www.pelvicpartnership.org.uk; 01235 820921

Pelvic, Obstetric and Gynaecological Physiotherapy: pogp.csp.org.uk

Pre-eclampsia: action-on-pre-eclampsia.org.uk; 020 8427 4217

Thrombosis: www.thrombosis-charity.org.uk; 0300 772 9603

Multiple births

Twins and Multiple Birth Association: www.tamba.org.uk; 0800 138 0509

Premature and poorly babies

Special care baby charity: www.bliss.org.uk; 0500 618 140

Relationships

Relate: www.relate.org.uk; 0300 100 1234

The Parent Connection: www.theparentconnection.org.uk

Safety

The Lullaby Trust: www.lullabytrust.org.uk

Child Accident Prevention Trust: www.capt.org.uk

Screening and abnormalities

Antenatal testing: www.arc-uk.org; 0845 077 2290

Group B Strep Support: www.gbss.org.uk; 01444 416 176

Information and support for Down's syndrome parents:
www.downs-syndrome.org.uk; 0333 1212 300

NHS Foetal Anomaly Screening Programme: www.gov.uk/topic/population-screening-programmes/fetal-anomaly

Support for lone parents

Campaigning charity: www.gingerbread.org.uk; 0808 802 0925

The Single Mum's Survival guide: www.thesinglemumssurvivalguide.co.uk

Index

Abdominal pain 27–8, 65

Acupuncture 168, 206, 273

Air travel 115

Alcohol 48, 60, 87–91, 247, 273

Amniocentesis 18

Amniotic fluid 18, 38, 51, 69, 75, 78, 79, 106, 123, 179, 207, 220

Amniotic sac 66, 74, 115,207

Anaemia 30–31, 35, 36, 38, 53, 179

Animals 115

Anomaly scan 15, 16, 79, 276

Antenatal care 9–13, 30, 94, 130, 131, 159, 179, 181–2

Antenatal classes 21–3, 161, 182

Antenatal notes 13, 201, 211, 269

Antenatal Results and Choices (ARC) 19–20

Antenatal supplements 30, 99, 110, 111–12

Antenatal tests 10, 13, 17–20, 41, 69, 276

Anxiety 29, 31–2. 60, 81, 104, 132, 169, 240

Aromatherapy 58, 114, 161, 168–9, 206, 273

Artificial sweeteners 103

Assisted delivery 222–3

Baby care 189–90. 248, 261–6, 275

Back pain 57–8, 60

Bearing down 217–18, 232

Birth partner 159, 160, 161, 163, 164, 171–3, 174, 192, 201, 213, 215, 216, 217, 220, 223, 225

Birth plan 153–80, 201, 216, 221, 223

Birthing pool 155, 156, 159, 161, 164, 168, 169, 173

Birthing unit 23, 254–6, 159, 172, 168, 169, 173, 201, 208, 212, 240, 269

Bleeding 15, 28–30, 66–7, 115, 118, 123, 146, 150, 176, 180, 210, 221, 251–2, 257

Bleeding gums (gingivitis) 34

Blood clot 35, 37, 176, 252, 258, 262

Blood pressure 11, 12, 41–2, 114, 115, 132, 182, 211, 213, 262

Blood sugar level 108

Bottle feeding 187–8, 197, 249–50

Braxton Hicks contractions 203, 208

Breasts (tender) 6, 255–6

Breastfeeding 71, 111, 183–8, 197, 220, 241–50, 252, 255, 274

Breast pads 185, 194, 196, 246

Breathlessness 31, 35

Breathing techniques 170–71, 192, 209, 211

Breech positions 84, 157, 174, 200

Bump 11, 58, 68–72, 116, 138, 194

Caesarean section 22, 256, 273

Emergency 67, 224–5

Planned/elective 174–8, 200
Recovery 258–9
Caffeine 39, 41, 48, 50, 61, 94–5
Carpal tunnel syndrome 53
Cervix (dilation) 213, 218
Chloasma 113
Chorionic villus sampling (CVS) 18
Colic 184, 264–6
Colostrum 33, 183, 194, 245
Colouring your hair 112–13
Constipation 27, 30, 35–6, 56, 62, 110, 117, 223, 254
Contractions 28, 144, 163–7, 171–2, 180, 195, 207–19, 252
Co-sleeping 189, 268, 275
Cramps 36, 204
Crying (baby) 264–6, 275

Dating scan 14–15, 17, 76
Deep vein thrombosis (DVT) 36
Dental care 24, 34
Depression (perinatal and postnatal) 31, 32, 43, 222, 269, 270
Diastasis recti 256
Diastasis symphysis pubis (DSP) 47
Diet (healthy) 35, 104–11
Dizziness 30, 62, 66, 114, 122, 133, 148, 257
Down's syndrome 17–19, 276
Driving 18
Drugs 21, 93–4, 165–7
Due date 8–9, 127, 203–4

Engagement 84, 201
Epidural 166–7, 221, 223, 225
Episiotomy 222–4, 252
Established labour 212–13
Estimated delivery date (EDD) 8–9, 14, 203

Exercise 36, 56, 57, 117–23, 119, 274
Exhaustion 6, 37–9, 44, 132, 193

Fainting 62, 66, 114, 122, 133, 137, 257
Fake tan and sunbeds 113, 257
Fetal alcohol syndrome 89
Folic acid 10, 110, 111
Food aversion 6, 39
Food cravings 6, 39, 105
Food safety 103, 104–5, 274
Forceps 177, 222, 261
Forgetfulness 32–3, 136

Gardening 114
Gas and air (entonox) 160, 163–4, 198
Gestational diabetes 69, 107–8, 205
Group B streptococcus 19–20, 276

Hairiness 39–40
Headaches 30, 40–42, 66, 94, 122, 167, 211, 257
Heartbeat (baby's) 11, 77, 113, 213–14, 224, 245
Heartburn 59–60, 93, 194
Home birth 156–8, 161, 165, 172, 273
Hot flush 61–2
Household chemicals and cleaning products 115
Hyperemesis gravidarum 45–6
Hypnobirthing 167, 169–70, 273

Incontinence 59
Indigestion 56, 59–60, 194
Induction 52, 204–5, 207, 214–15
Infections 12, 30, 35, 49–51, 67, 91, 95–6, 97, 114, 117, 150, 175, 176,

177, 179, 207, 211, 251, 253, 257
Insomnia 31, 38, 40, 60–61, 94, 132, 146, 194
Itching 49, 51–2, 55, 62, 66, 194, 223, 252, 254, 259

Keeping in touch (KIT) days 139
Kicking 63, 66, 78

Labour 67, 149, 162–73, 180, 182, 195, 197–8, 205–21
Lanugo (hair) 77, 82, 261
Listeria 97, 99, 102
Low milk supply 248

Massage 34, 58, 148, 160, 171, 217
Mastitis 249, 255
Maternity Allowance 128
Maternity clothes 70–2
Maternity leave 125–30, 139, 140, 190
    Ordinary Maternity Leave (OML) 127, 140
    Shared parental leave 129
Maternity pads 251, 253, 254
Maternity pay 128, 130, 140
Membrane sweep 204
Metallic taste 5, 6
Miscarriage 18, 29–30, 67, 89, 91, 93, 94, 96, 116, 150, 275
Mood swings 42–3
Morning sickness 6, 43–6, 48, 94, 105, 134–5
Mucus 148, 150, 251
Multiple births 178, 276

Nasal congestion 40, 53
Nausea 6, 43–6, 134–5

National Childbirth Trust (NCT) 21–2, 161, 274, 275
Natural birth 22, 156, 172, 160–62
Nipples 6, 55, 149, 185, 186, 206, 242, 243, 249
Nosebleeds 53
Nuchal translucency screening 17–18
Nursing bra 185, 196

Obstetrician 10, 82, 154, 173, 174, 178, 222, 224, 275
Obstetric cholestasis 52, 194, 275
Oedema 194
Overheating 61–2, 114

Pain in the hands 53–4
Pain relief 58, 158, 159, 161, 162–71, 204, 222, 223, 225, 258
Paint 114
Paternity rights 129–30
Pilates 46, 119, 256
Pelvic floor 59, 119, 120–21, 177, 223, 253, 257
Pelvic pain 46–7, 133, 193
Perineum 194–5, 218, 219, 223, 252
Period cramps 209, 210
Pethidine 161, 165–6
Piles (haemorrhoids) 62–3, 254
Placenta 18, 38, 42, 44, 69, 74–5, 89
    Abruption 67
    Delivery 159, 212, 220, 221–2
    Low-lying 15
    Praevia 15, 67
    Retained 221
Position
    Baby's 11, 15, 18, 69, 82, 84, 157, 174, 178, 200–201, 213

Birthing 158, 159, 192, 215–16, 218
Postpartum haemorrhage (PPH) 221
Pre-eclampsia 12, 41–2, 65, 106, 157, 194, 205, 276
Premature labour/birth 50, 89, 91, 97, 115, 144, 178–9, 268, 276
Public transport 137
Pushing 165, 166, 167, 211–12, 217–19, 221

Raspberry leaf tea 195, 206
Reflexology 169, 206, 274
Relationship with your partner 23, 151–2, 276
Restless leg syndrome 47–8
Returning to work 140–41
Rib pain 63, 194
Rupture of membranes 179

Safe sleeping 267–8
Salmonella 98, 99, 100
Saunas, hot tubs, steam baths and Jacuzzis 62, 113–14
Sex during pregnancy 67, 120, 143–50, 206, 253
Sex of baby 16–17
Shared parental leave 129–30, 274
Skin changes 6, 40, 51, 54–5, 110, 113, 194
Skin-to-skin 160, 219–20, 245
Sleep 41, 42, 47–8, 60–61, 132–3, 192
Smell, heightened sense of 6, 48–9
Smoking 91–2, 268, 273
Spotting 7, 28, 66–7
Stitches 220, 223, 252–4, 259, 262
Stress 40, 104, 131, 132, 137

Stretch marks 64–5, 257
Swollen feet and hands 64–5, 194
Syntocinon 215

TENS machine 164–5
Thrombosis 37, 276
Thrush 49, 67
Tokophobia 176
Tongue tie 183, 246, 248–9
Toxoplasmosis 96, 97, 99, 114–15

Ultrasound scans 9, 13–18, 69, 76, 79
Umbilical cord 75, 78, 160, 220, 261
Urinary tract infection (UTI) 50
Urinating (frequency) 49–50

Vacuum extraction (ventouse) 155, 218, 222, 261
Vaginal bleeding 7, 15, 28–9, 65, 66–7, 115, 123, 146, 150, 180, 210, 221, 251–52, 257
Vaginal discharge 49, 50–51, 67, 203, 251
Varicose veins 55–6
Vernix 78, 220, 261

Waters 150, 179–80, 205, 206, 207, 211, 212, 215
Weight
  Mother's 12, 38, 45, 55, 57, 64, 68, 69, 105–8, 111, 184, 193
  Baby's 19, 73, 84, 89, 91, 93, 94, 103, 260
Wind 27, 56–7, 259

X-rays 116